I0421389

Detoxify Your Body, Lose Weight, Get Healthy & Transform Your Life Volumes 1-3

Volume 1 - The 10-Day 'At-Home' Colon Cleansing Formula

Volume 2 - Bug Off! A 30-Day Parasite, Liver, Kidney Detox & Weight Loss Plan

Volume 3 - Lose 30 Pounds in 30 Days (Or More) With Intermittent Fasting & At-Home Coffee Enemas

ROBERT DAVE JOHNSTON

Published by:

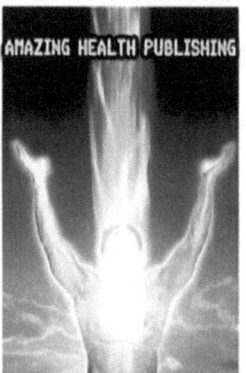

If you are interested in reading the next volume,
follow Rob on Twitter @RobDaveJohnston

Copyright

Copyright © 2012, Robert Dave Johnston, Amazing Health Publishing. Cover and internal design © Robert Dave Johnston. All rights reserved. No part of this book may be reproduced in any form or by any electronic or mechanical means including information storage and retrieval systems – except in the case of brief quotations in articles or reviews – without the permission in writing from its publisher, Amazing Horror Publishing/Robert Dave Johnston. All of the people, places and things depicted in this book are fictional. Any resemblance to a real person, place or otherwise is totally coincidental.

Disclaimer & Legal Notices

The health-related information and suggestions contained in any of the books or written material mentioned above are based on the research, experience and opinions of the Author and other contributors. Nothing herein should be misinterpreted as actual medical advice, such as one would obtain from a Physician, or as advice for self-diagnosis or as any manner of prescription for self-treatment.

Neither is any information herein to be considered a particular or general cure for any ailment, disease or other health issue. The material contained within is offered strictly and solely for the purpose of providing Holistic health education to the general public. Persons with any health condition should consult a medical professional before entering this or any fasting, weight loss, detoxification or health related program.

Even if you suffer from no known illness, we recommend that you seek medical advice before starting any fasting, weight loss and/or detoxification program, and before choosing to follow any advice given this book. For any products or services mentioned or suggested in this book, you should read all packaging and instructions, as no substance, natural or drug, can be guaranteed to work in everyone.

Information and statements regarding dietary supplements, products or services mentioned in this book many not have been evaluated by the Food and Drug Administration and are not intended to diagnose, treat, cure, or prevent any disease. Never disregard or delay in seeking professional medical advice because of something you have read in this book.

Nothing that you read in this book should be regarded as medical or health advice. If you do anything recommended in this book, without the supervision of a licensed medical doctor, you do so at your own risk. Not recommended for persons with any health related condition unless supervised by a qualified health practitioner.

Because there is always some risk involved in any health-related program, the Author, Publisher and contributors assume no responsibility for any adverse effects or consequences resulting from the use of any suggested preparations or procedures described in any of the books or other written materials associated with the website FitnessThroughFasting.com. The author reserves the right to alter and update his opinions based on new conditions at any time.

Dedication

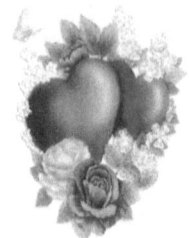

This series of books are dedicated to my mother Sonia Noemi, without whom I would not even be alive today. I love you mom. Thank you for never losing faith in me and supporting me, even when everything seemed hopeless and everyone else had given up on me. I owe you everything. I could collect all of the precious stones on this earth and lay them on your lap, and even still, I would not even come close to giving back to you all that you have given me.

Volume 1
The 10-Day 'At-Home' Colon Cleansing Formula

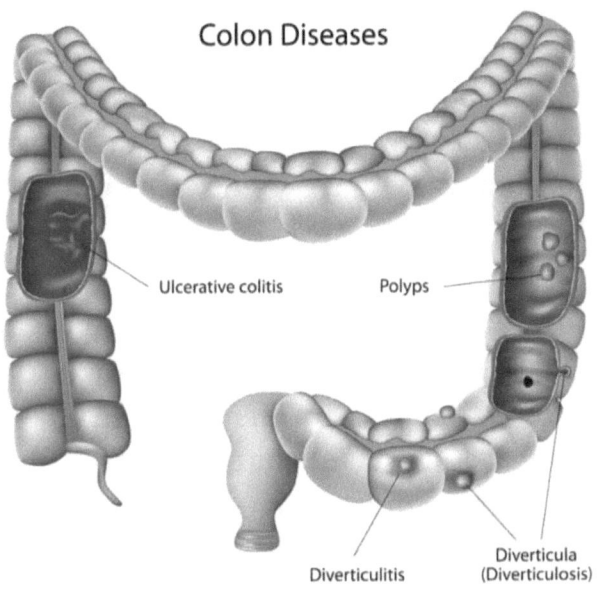

Colon Diseases

Ulcerative colitis   Polyps

Diverticulitis   Diverticula (Diverticulosis)

"By picking up this book, you are making drastic changes in your life. Change requires vision, sacrifice and determination. There is, however, something you must keep very clear in your mind: *The benefits of sticking to your guns and following through with this process are monumental and life-changing.*"

Chapter 1
The Challenge of
Detoxification

If you have never done a colon cleanse before, then I salute you: You are about to give your body a tremendous gift that will help you to eliminate toxic, disease-causing waste that may have been curtailing your health for a long time.

I know of one man who, during a cleanse, eliminated several pounds of rotten, undigested meat from his colon. And, to be sure, examples like that abound. In this book, I am going to give you a simple and straightforward method to achieve ultimate colon cleansing, from the comfort of your own home. I struggled with liver and colon toxicity for many years; in fact, at one point it got so bad that I thought my days were numbered. But by being consistent as well as patient, I was able to turn my health around, and that has happened to a great extent thanks to the colon cleansing remedy presented here. I was far gone physically; a morbidly obese, self-destructive basket case.

If this can work for someone like me (*who reached low bottoms of food addiction and obesity*), then by all means I believe that it will do wonders for you as well.

Rectal Phobia

I know that any procedure involving the rectum will never be on anyone's *Top 10* list of '*Most Wanted.*' It took me years to let go of my prejudice against colon cleansing; that is, until I reached a point of desperation and became willing to do it – **FOR MYSELF**. If you feel resistant to colon cleansing because it involves (more than usual) anal discharging and feces, please get over it.

How would your house be if you put the trash on bags but never took them out? Can you imagine the stench, cockroaches and filth that would result? The same happens with our bodies. When the colon is strained from poor and/or excessive eating, a lot of the debris that is supposed to go out lingers, rotting and intoxicating the bloodstream, which, in turn, adversely affects the functioning of vital organs – even the brain. If you can see it from that perspective, it will be easier to get through the resistance. I'm certain that you do not want toxic trash circulating around your body creating havoc. Once you take action, you will begin to see colon cleansing in a whole new light.

Persistence and Patience

And I am very glad that I did. Within a few days of my first cleanse, I started to feel lighter, more energized and my mood swings, which had become very volatile and painful, began to stabilize. The key is persistence and patience. Persistence in taking the action, and patience in allowing the body to do what it does 'at its pace.' I say this because many people write to tell me that, "they did a colon cleanse and nothing came out." Well, imagine if a soft piece of clay is permitted to harden and become as tough as a rock. How many times will you have to pound the rock with a pick before it finally comes apart? The same is the case with our bodies.

If you have eaten poorly for a long time, or even if you haven't, chances are that you will need to be patient and try, try again if the initial cleansing doesn't produce the desired results. Please... I am begging you: Take the action, but be patient and good to your body. It will **ALWAYS** produce the outcomes you desire, IF you are long-suffering and unrelenting. And by no means increase the dosages in this colon cleanse formula, even if at first you do not see much discharge. Keep working at it, follow my instructions, and – eventually- it will happen. That has been my experience over the years, and I am certain that you, too, will achieve great things through this type of cleanse.

Home Remedy
Vs. Cleansing Kits

I have put this book together so that it is short and to-the-point. I give you a list of ingredients that you will need for the "at-home" cleansing remedy. If you do not have time to prepare these home remedies, or if you simply do not wish to delve into the matter that deeply, I have also included links to equivalent *"cleansing kits."* However, I strongly encourage you to take the time and learn to prepare the home remedy. Having that type of holistic knowledge (*knowing how to detox your body*) is invaluable. No matter where you may find yourself, you will be able to put together a home colon-cleanse remedy. The ingredients are available at your local supermarket, health food store or herb/produce vendor.

Note: None of what we are doing here is easy. You are making drastic changes in your life. Change requires vision, sacrifice and determination. There is, however, something you must keep very clear in your mind: "*The benefits of sticking to your guns and following through with this process are monumental and life-changing*". Clarify and expand your goals. Write in a journal what your goals are in relation to your health. Remind yourself **DAILY** exactly why you want to detoxify and improve your health.

You will feel great pride and self-esteem when following through until you accomplish your goals. These positive feelings will last much longer than the piece of chocolate cake you are reaching for. Now is the time! Stop giving up and returning to your old ways. Remember: **A minute on the lips, forever on the hips!**

Chapter 2
Constipation

There is an old saying that you have to: "exhale before you can inhale". Put another way, it is necessary to empty before one can fill. The same applies to the colon. You have to drain what is inside before you can nourish. You can eat all the health-food in the world, but if your colon is clogged and polluted, the benefit will be paltry. That is the "why" of colon cleansing.

One of the most frequent problems people experience today is constipation. A constipated system is one in which the transition time of toxic waste is slow. The longer the "*transit time*," the longer the toxic matter sits in the bowel. This allows the waste to putrefy, ferment and – even worse - be reabsorbed into the blood stream.

The longer your body has putrefying food in the intestines, the greater the risk of developing disease. **Did you know?** -> Even if you have one bowel movement per day, you could still have several meals worth of waste-matter in your colon! I don't know about you, but that does **NOT** sound very pleasant.

Bowel movements are the basis of human health. If you don't have at least **ONE** bowel movement per day, then you are probably walking towards disease. Anatomically-speaking, the human body has not changed much over the past millennia. But, the food that we eat has. Refined sugar, white flour, hormone/antibiotic-filled meats and saturated fats have literally taken over the daily diet - especially in the US. This type of highly-processed food causes great harm to the digestive system. It also keeps the body addicted. I just finished a great book called "The End of Overeating" by Dr. David Kessler. In it, he goes into great detail in his coverage of the fast food industry and the American diet. I encourage you to read it.

If your diet has been less than optimum, then all congestion and toxins must be removed. This begins with colon cleansing, and here's the bottom line: One of the greatest challenges our bodies face is the effective removal of wastes and toxins. As the colon becomes impacted with putrefied waste, its shape can stretch like a balloon and develop Diverticulitis – a dangerous condition of inflammation which can become infected. In advanced cases, prolonged constipation and straining could even lead to Rectal Prolapse.

Chapter 3
Is Your Colon Healthy?

If you are experiencing any of the symptoms listed below, then your digestive system is probably **<u>NOT</u>** in the best of health. You may have an unhealthy colon if you:

* Have infrequent bowel movements or very small amounts. Small pellet-shaped stools are a common indication that something is wrong.

*Need to strain to eliminate. The toilet is no place to get an "abdominal workout". Effortless and quick bowel movements are key signs of a healthy colon.

* Require a substantial amount of time to go. If you have a 500-page novel next to the toilet as opposed to the newspaper, that may be a clue!

When I visited a friend recently and saw a copy of "War and Peace" in the bathroom, I knew he needed a colon cleanse. This book will focus on an "at-home" colon cleansing system I learned years ago when I struggled with a toxic liver. It is very powerful and can be used any time your digestion is sluggish, you feel heavy, congested or lethargic - or when you are coming down with a cold.

Headaches, bad breath, white coat on the tongue, bloating and constant flatulence are all indicators that it is time for a colon cleanse. So keep this book handy. You can use it in the future or pass it on to a loved-one who may need it!

Important Reminder

Constipation and other bowel disorders can be a sign of a serious condition. If you find that you do not have a bowel movement in spite of this cleanse, then I strongly encourage you to see your doctor at once. A variety of diseases can cause irregularity of the bowels.

Disease often begins with a toxic bowel. Fewer bowel movements harbor a potentially-fertile breeding ground for sickness. Infrequent or poor quality bowel movements over an extended period of time can be hazardous to your health.

LIKEWISE,

Use Common Sense! Discontinue this colon-cleanse if you experience persistent diarrhea for longer than two days. Drink at least half-a-gallon of water daily while on this cleanse. If you are more than 20 pounds overweight, as much as three days of diarrhea may be normal, especially if you have never done a cleanse before. If you are NOT overweight, then you must be vigilant and follow your instinct when doing this type of cleanse.

Chapter 4
Pre-Cleanse Preparation

If you have been eating poorly and/or excessively, your colon cleansing efforts will go a lot further if you prepare your body. And that means removing from your diet any and all junk, greasy and sugary foods that you are accustomed to eating. The removal of these toxic foods will send your body into ultimate detoxification mode, and it will work hard on your behalf to eliminate the filth that keeps you from experiencing optimal health and wellness.

Of course, usual offenders that must be eliminated (at least during the ten-day colon cleanse) are sugars, starches (enriched flour) and saturated fats. These include but are not limited to pastries, candy, white rice, white bread, soda pops, butter, frying oil, cheeseburgers, pizza, etc...For further guidance, here is a list of 'banned foods.' Stay away from then during the ten-day cleanse.

I'd love it if you stayed away from them permanently, as your health, energy and overall wellness would shoot off the charts if you did. However, for the sake of this immediate cleanse, you are to abstain from all of the foods listed below during the 10-day period.

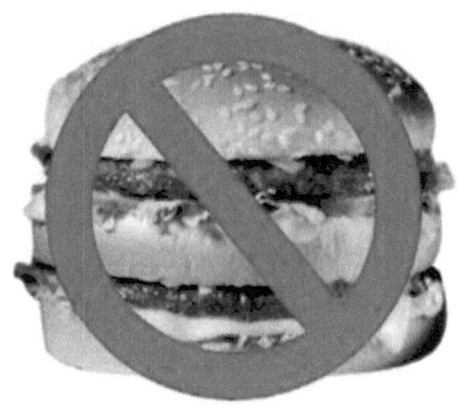

Banned Foods

*Salt - you get plenty of it from the foods that you eat. When I first started my diet years ago, I was kind of shocked to see that salt was banned. I spoke against it actually. I have come to realize that the foods we eat all have sodium, and that a healthy adult really has no need for 'salt' except to make the food taste better. In addition, when I stopped using salt, I immediately dropped like 15 pounds. It was mostly water weight, but it showed me that I was retaining a LOT of liquids, and that was greatly due to my abuse of salt and seasonings.

* **Sugar** - absolute trash, toxic to the body... good for nothing - stay away! I could write pages and pages about sugar. I am sure that you yourself can admit that this is one of our greatest (if not our greatest) enemy. I mean it. Enemy. Any prolonged return to sugar will, sooner or later, result in full-blown intoxication of the bloodstream and digestive system.

I don't kid myself by thinking that "I'm cured." I still am susceptible to sugar and to binging. What keeps me free and clean is **NOT** to put sugar into my body... period. I can't draw the same conclusion for you, but I am certain that you probably have your own stories to tell about sugar and how it has affected your weight, life and health.

* **Fried Foods** - Absolute filthy grease fest that leads to obesity and other diseases.

* **Cheese** - Cheese is great but it has way too much fat. For the time being, steer clear. Later on, once you finish the cleanse, you

will be able to have treats from time to time. So don't let the mind start telling you that your 'life is over' because you can't eat this or that. Just tell the mind to shut up and keep moving forward. Works like a charm for me.

* **Dairy Products** - dairy has a lot of fat, is high in sugar content and has been known to cause digestive system inflammation. But I'm not totally heartless. Stick to non-fat milk, how's that? Anything above non-fat is banned.

* **Red Meat** - I personally don't have anything against red meat. In fact, I have been known to eat a piece of meat on rare occasion. Right now, we are banning it because it has a lot of fat, and because I want your digestive system to be given easy food to digest. Later on you can have a piece of meat here and there if you want. Right now... it's banned.

* **Alcohol** - Alcohol is packed with empty calories. Calories with **ZERO** nutritional value. And booze turns to sugar. Bad all over. If you drink frequently, cut it down to a minimum. You're doing this for your

health and to reach a goal that is important to **YOU**. If you have to go a few days without drinking, your arm is not going to fall off. You'll live. A cup of wine with dinner is fine, but nothing more than that at this juncture.

* **Butter or Margarine** - As they say in New York, "Forget about it!!!" Butter and margarine are pure fat and we don't want it.

* **Fruit Juices** - If you read the label of most orange juice brands, you will see that the sugar content is through the roof. Yes, it is natural sugar, but sugar nonetheless. You can have one glass of juice in the morning, but you need to water it down 50/50. Drinking straight juice at this phase is basically like injecting blubber directly into your belly. Stay away. Drink veggie juice instead...but make sure that it is the low sodium veggie juice. :-)

***White Enriched Bread** - That stuff is like dropping a ball of cement into the stomach. White flour, doughy garbage really is terrible for human health. I was going to ban all breads, but I remembered that the Ezekiel brand (green bag) is actually very good. You can eat one slice here and there as partial replacement to your carbohydrate servings. We'll get into all of that in just a minute.

*Junk Food of ANY Kind - I think that it definitely goes without saying that junk food is out. And not just out for a little while. Hopefully, it is out of your life for good. That crap is like wearing a ball and chain. It enslaves us to cravings that are never satisfied and only get stronger and more violent.

Foods to Limit List:

*Fruits (Stick To Strawberries or Cantaloupe)
* Tomatoes
* Peas or Corn
* Olive Oil

Starting immediately, eliminate **ALL** of these foods and beverages from your diet... period.

This is the beginning of the process. For now, continue to eat whatever else you have been eating **EXCEPT** for the foods that are listed above. I want you to take a full step forward and discontinue eating any and all junk. That's the whole point of our work together, right? To help you achieve measurable improvements in your health. So cut it all out. Do not eat <u>even a little</u> of them anymore. I mean <u>Nothing</u>, <u>No More</u>, <u>Finito</u>, <u>Nada</u>!

You are taking the <u>monumental</u> step of removing **ALL** toxic foods from your diet. I use the word *'monumental'* because, in truth, you are now in the minority. The majority of people live their whole lives and **NEVER** confront their eating behaviors as you are now doing. And since you won't be dumping more and more crap into your belly, the colon cleansing remedy will be able to focus on the breakdown and discharge of existing debris.

Chapter 5
Eat Six Times Daily

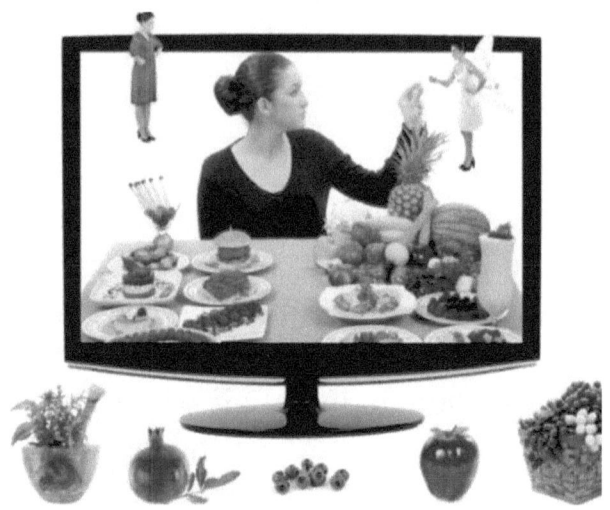

Eating smaller meals with greater frequency, totaling six meals per day, is one of the strategies that helped me to expel the most intestinal debris through colon cleansing. I would strongly encourage you to observe the banned foods list during the 10-day colon cleanse, as well as change your eating structure to one of six smaller meals.

This method will accelerate your metabolism, meaning that the body can process and expel toxins faster and more efficiently. But, don't worry... this doesn't have to be hard.

The six-meals-per-day structure includes breakfast, mid-morning snack, lunch, mid-afternoon snack, dinner and evening snack. The metabolism is like a fire. Let me give you an analogy to illustrate.

Imagine that you were stranded in a very cold place and need to keep a fire burning to survive the night. Would you be better off dumping a huge amount of firewood at once, or would the fire burn longer and keep you warmer if you added small amounts of wood frequently? Of course, the answer is the latter. The more frequently you eat (observing the banned foods list), the better you will feel and the more energy you will have.

Consequently, the metabolism will work evenly and continuously, which results in faster weight loss and elimination of toxins. Having larger meals with less frequency is like dumping a large amount of wood into the fire. You will get one heck of blaze initially, but it will die out sooner and not provide as much heat (energy) as it would if you added wood more sparingly.

This is what causes the monster cravings that keep people trapped in binging and overeating for years. If you want to disconnect the cravings and succeed in your colon cleansing, eat more frequently.

To help you see how this works, here is a sample menu from a typical day in my life:

Sample Menu

Breakfast 8:00 AM

1 Cup of Oatmeal with 1 Cup Skim Milk, a Handful of Raisins or Plums
Three Egg Whites mixed with, 3 OZ Ground Turkey
1 Cup of Green Tea with Stevia

Mid-Morning Snack 10AM

1 Apple or Pear Mixed With One Cup of Nonfat Yogurt (Plain)
OR, ONE Apple, Pear, Banana or Other Fruit

Lunch - Noon

Big salad with lettuce, tomato and other veggies you may like. For dressing, use olive oil (no more than 1 teaspoon) and balsamic vinegar.
1 Envelope of Low-Sodium Tuna
1 4OZ Baked Potato or Sweet Potato

Mid-Afternoon Snack 3PM

Same as before - I usually have a piece of fruit mixed with yogurt. At this time in the afternoon, I also drink another cup of green tea. Green tea has energy-boosting and body-heating properties. It will help to give you a pep as well as calm hunger pangs. In addition to green tea, seltzer water (sparkling water/club soda) is great to navigate hunger.

Dinner - 6PM

Six-to-eight ounces of chicken, fish or ground turkey (I like to make turkey patties)
Large salad as the one eaten for lunch

Steamed Broccoli, Cauliflower and Carrots (most supermarkets have prepackaged vegetable combinations that are ready to steam and eat).
4OZ Baked Potato or Sweet Potato OR 4OZ of Whole Wheat or Whole Grain Pasta OR 4 OZ of Brown Rice

Evening Snack - 8PM

Big salad with 3OZ Chicken, Fish or Ground Turkey - No carbohydrates.
A piece of fruit with Non-fat Yogurt
Cup of Chamomile Tea - Chamomile tea is great to drink at night because it will help soothe hunger as well as calm you and get you ready for bed.

You should not eat anything at least two hours prior to turning in. Sometimes I also take one 500 mg tablet of Tryptophan at night to help me sleep.

Tryptophan is an awesome amino acid that helps to stabilize mood. At this point I'm done eating for the day and drink only water until 8AM the following morning.

Again ->

NEVER EAT FOR THE LAST TWO
HOURS BEFORE YOU GO TO BED.

Do you ingest a large portion of your daily calories a few hours before bedtime?

When your body is at rest, all of your metabolic processes slow down so you don't burn as many calories as you would during the day while you are actively moving around. When you eat large portions of food shortly before you go to bed, many of those calories are going to be stored as fat.

Unfortunately, some people eat very few calories all day long, then gulp down a large dinner – and then munch on snacks all evening before they go to bed! Throughout the day they may have ingested 500 to 700 calories, and then 2,000 to 3,000 calories right before they go to bed. Bad idea! Tape your mouth shut if you have to. But eat no more!

Chapter 6
Home Colon Cleansing

Alright, let's take a look at the ingredients you will need to prepare your home colon cleansing formula. Each of the ingredients listed below are the very same that I use to prepare my own colon cleansing remedy. After years of frequent colon cleansings, even with at-home colonic kits, these products are the ones that produce the very best results. You can order them online and they should arrive in roughly two days.

Alternatively, you can browse for them in your local health food store or supermarket. I like Amazon because, in 99% of the cases, the prices are notably lower, and the shipping is fast. At the bottom of the list you will note that I mention the Lifiber colon cleansing kit as an alternative. As I said earlier, go with the kit only if you absolutely, positively do not have the time or disposition to prepare the remedy.

My suggestion is that you definitely use the remedy, get acquainted with it and master it. You don't know if a kit will be around at a time of need, while the basic ingredients in the remedy are easily found pretty much everywhere. Once you get comfortable preparing the remedy and **SEE** the amazing results, there's no doubt that this kind of holistic medicine will stay in your family for the long-term.

Colon Cleanse Formula Ingredients

Organic Apple Juice - Apple juice helps the body fight-off bad cholesterol while enhancing cardiovascular health. It also combats constipation, cleans the liver and kidneys and is known to boost intestinal/colon health.

Apple Cider Vinegar - Diminishes sinus infections, effectively treats skin conditions such as acne, boosts the immune system, speeds-up the metabolism and promotes weight loss.

Helps to improve digestion and relieves constipation, can help fight-off the development of bladder stones and urinary tract infections.

It also relieves symptoms associated with gout and arthritis.

Aloe Vera Juice (NOT "Drink") Aids digestion, promotes weight loss, decreases blood sugar levels, boosts the immune system.

Psyllium Husk Powder (*Preferably Unflavored*) - Constipation Relief. Psyllium Husk Powder is a bulk laxative highly effective in the treatment of constipation.

When ingested, the powder absorbs water and turns into a gelatinous ball inside the digestive system. As it expands, jellylike ball pushes waste products out of the colon by force, triggering what can often be massive bowel movements.

Furthermore, Psyllium has lubricating properties which facilitate the passage of stool, thus reducing pain in cases of chronic hemorrhoids or colitis.

Psyllium also treats diarrhea by absorbing extra water in the digestive tract and helping to make stools firm.

Cascara Sagrada -> **Cascara Sagrada** is a herbal laxative which is retrieved from the reddish bark of the Pacific Northwest native three, Rhamnus purshiana.

Liquid Chlorophyll - helps the body to flush out toxic heavy metals such as mercury. Liquid Chlorophyll assists in the removal of germs as well as thwarts the growth of new ones. Boosts digestive system functions.

Average Cost of This Remedy -> $50

OR, ONE, MAYBE TWO LiFiber Colon Detox Kits @ app. $65.95 each. Of the few 'cleansing kits' that I've used over the years, this LiFiber is, by far, the strongest and most complete. If you choose to go this path, make sure to read the instructions on the box before starting. Overall, the Lifiber would be taken at night just like the remedy.

The difference here is that all you need to add is water. It isn't necessary to mix various ingredients as is the case with the traditional remedy. Still, I vote in favor of the remedy because it places at your fingertips a very powerful remedy that will always get the job done. It may seem like a drudgery at first to mix this with that and that. But once you get used to it, you will hopefully come to love it as much as I do.

*I Recommend That You Do This 10-Day Colon Cleanse Again in TWO Months as Follow up, and Then At least Once Annually Thereafter.

Chapter 7
Preparing the Remedy

Once you have purchased all of the items, make some room in the kitchen counter so that you can work, setting aside any appliances or other objects that will get in the way. Bottom line: give yourself plenty of counter space. Get a used towel, one that you aren't particularly fond of, and lay it on top of the counter. Take out all of the ingredients and line them up around the towel. In addition, you will need a 16-ounce plastic or glass cup in which to mix the ingredients. Some people prefer to wear gloves when preparing these remedies; that's left totally to your discretion.

Add into the 16-ounce cup:

.

•1 heaping teaspoon Psyllium Husk Powder - (preferably unflavored)

•1/2 cup organic, unfiltered (preferably raw or unpasteurized) apple juice – if you cannot find raw apple juice, then pasteurized is acceptable if you add a tablespoon of Apple Cider Vinegar.

•2 tablespoons Chlorophyll.

•2 capsules of Cascara Sagrada - herbal laxative. Simply open the capsule and dump the brownish powder into the glass.

•2 tablespoons Aloe Vera Juice – make sure to get juice, not drink. Aloe Vera drinks are mostly water and NOT what we are looking for here.

•A 12-ounce glass of water.

Mix vigorously for 30 seconds and down the hatch! Drink the colon-cleansing formula nightly **TWO** hours before going to bed. Make sure to drink it right-away after you mix it because Psyllium bulks up quickly. After you drink the first glass, there will nearly-always be residue. Refill the glass with water, stir the contents and drink up until **ALL** of the contents are gone. Do this every night for the next **TEN** days.

Belly Massage

Many times, the intestinal debris in our bodies is very hard and stubborn, not wanting to let go of the walls of the colon. Spend as much time as possible massaging your stomach with both hands –covering the left, right, bottom and upper parts of the abdomen. Pay close attention to your liver. Play some music and let it sink in; visualize toxins, parasites and hardened fecal matter being expelled from your body.

Take as much time as needed in this process. I once had a female friend step on my stomach and move her foot all around the belly. She didn't put ALL of her weight on my stomach; just enough to exert some pressure. And, to my amazement, five minutes later I was sprinting to the toilet and ended up expelling a huge, black rock of debris that I'm certain had been inside of me for years. Really, really work it!

For some people with large levels of toxicity, the evacuation process can be dramatic and almost immediate. If that is the case for you, go ahead and eliminate. You may feel cramps in your stomach and some abdomen pain. This is fairly normal for most people. Make sure to look at the discharge once you are done. What color is it? Is it really dark or even black?

If so, then it is likely that you are making good progress. If at any time you see blood in the stool, stop the cleanse immediately and go see your doctor at once!

Chapter 8
Assignments

1. **Purchase ALL of the Ingredients Needed to Complete the Entire 10-day Colon Cleanse.** It will be much more beneficial to have all of the ingredients handy, so you can focus on the daily preparation and consumption, NOT on having to go out shopping because you forgot or did not get an ingredient. Seriously, step one is to get all of the ingredients... every single one of them. THEN you can come back home and start preparation

2. **Drink the Colon Cleanse remedy for 10 days, strictly adhering to the banned foods we looked at earlier.** When hunger and/or cravings come around to hassle you, drink two large glasses of water and breathe. Spend time writing about your health-related goals. Fill your mind with the powerful reasons why you want to accomplish this detox cleanse, and in which way will your life be improved with total body detoxification.

The cost of this cleansing process is minimal in comparison to the huge health benefits that you will receive, not to mention added quality years of life!

3. **Stay Close to and Communicate with at least one person that you trust who will support you in this task and not judge.**

Any type of detox cleansing is initially going to be challenging, so it helps a lot to have someone standing by to give you a hand and cheer you on. So don't be a Lone Ranger please.

This step is designed to give you ongoing "human" support. Human support will prove invaluable to you during this cleanse. Go to Fitness Through Fasting's - - Fasting Forum and post messages. Ask for a buddy! Read other people's posts and reach out! You will find many others on the same path. You may even make life-long friends!

When tempted to stray, always remember: Nothing Tastes as Good as Thin Feels!

God bless and Godspeed,

ROBERT DAVE JOHNSTON

Volume 2:
Bug Off! A 30-Day Parasite, Liver, Kidney Detox & Weight Loss Plan

Important Reminder

The body detoxification recipes presented in this book can, in some cases, cause unpleasant symptoms. This "curative crisis" is part of the process of restoring the body's overall balance and usually goes away on its own after a few days.

However, if you suffer from a chronic illness or are taking prescription medications, it is strongly suggested that you see your doctor **BEFORE** carrying out any type of detoxification program.

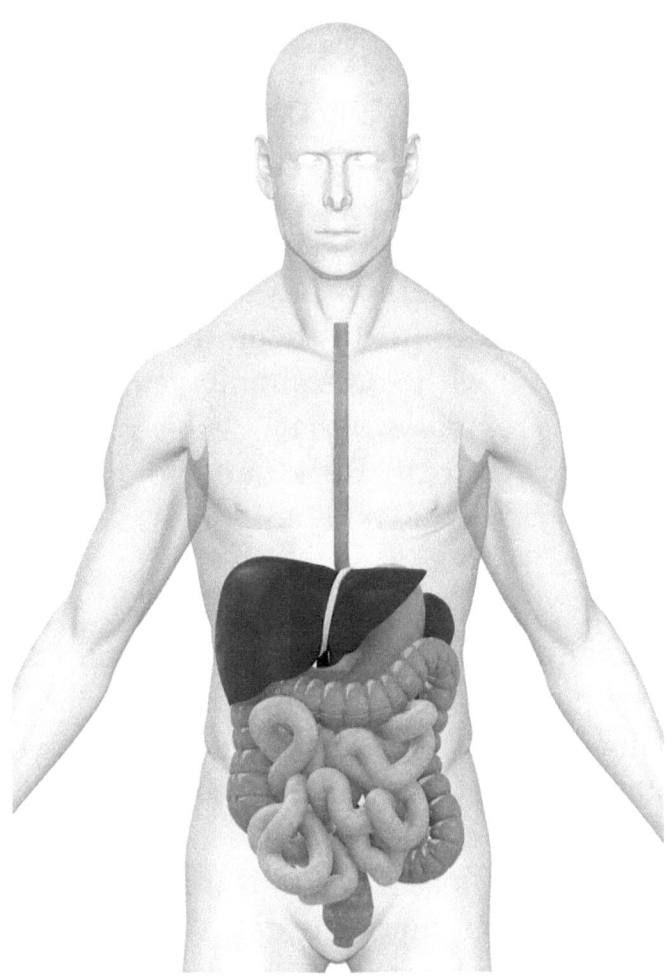

"The body detox program you are about to embark on has the power to transform your life in ways that you cannot even imagine. Yes, there may be some discomfort. But whatever discomfort you go through is **NOTHING** in comparison to the huge health benefits that you will gain."

Chapter 1:
Total Body Detox in 30 Days

Welcome to your cleansing and healing journey. You have taken a very important step toward optimum physical, mental and spiritual health. In this book, I am going to present you with some simple yet powerful holistic remedies that will help to thoroughly detoxify the kidneys and liver, as well as rid your body of disease-causing parasites.

Furthermore, I will outline a simple diet (together with sample menus and list of banned foods) that I highly recommend you follow during the entire detox process. If you observe these dietary instructions, you can expect to lose 20 pounds (or more) in 30 days, the duration of the detox process. So I want you to be ready to do some work, and to do it soon – **without procrastination**.

I can assure you that, if you follow through with this material to the very best of your ability, you are going to see some measurable (*even dramatic*) improvements in your health (as well as notable weight loss). The important part is that you <u>take</u> <u>action</u>. I want to motivate you to **dive into this process with all of your might**. You will not be disappointed by the results, I promise. You will learn how to prepare powerful home remedies that will place sickness against the ropes, and a simple diet that can help you to lose **A LOT** of weight. It is my hope that you will this material for many years to come. You can even teach them to your loved ones!

Ok. Here's how this is going to work:

Initially, I will encourage you to make some diet adjustments for at least 7-10 days prior to starting the detox process. If you have been eating poorly or in excess, following a pre-detox cleansing diet is indispensable to maximize results. Once that initial cleansing-diet phase is completed, we will place our emphasis on kidney/gall bladder cleansing for **<u>FIVE</u>** days.

You'll then rest for a full 24-hour, from where we'll launch the **30-day** parasite elimination phase. Finally, I'll give you detailed instructions on how to detox your liver in **16-24 hours**. I want you to enjoy the benefits of detox cleansing for the long term. Therefore, improving your eating habits is going to be very important.

As I said before: please don't procrastinate. You purchased this book because you want to optimize your health and increase quality of life. It is imperative that you pick a start day and make a firm commitment with yourself that you **WILL** get this done. I realize that, if you are new to detox cleansing, a lot of this material may be a bit intimidating or overwhelming.

I also want you to be aware that, depending on your health and level of toxicity, you are likely to experience some physical discomfort. But any discomfort that you go through with this cleanse is **NOTHING** in comparison to the huge health benefits that you stand to gain.

Discomfort means that the body is healing, that it is eliminating trash that was harming you. o please keep that in mind as we walk through the program.

Don't worry, I will be here to guide you and motivate you all the way.

I have gone through this process many times and will give you everything that I've got. I care and want you to succeed.

So let's dive right in and talk about the pre-cleanse diet adjustments.

Chapter 2:
Weight Loss & Detox Cleansing Diet

There is no question: the results that you produce from this detox program will be **GREATER** if you adjust your diet a few days before starting and, at the very least, during the process. You want to help your body as much as possible with detoxification. What you eat (and not eat) will make a tremendous difference.

Of course, I want you to improve your eating habits permanently. **THAT** is what will truly transform your life and health. As I said, I will give you a list of foods that you should definitely avoid. Mostly, I am referring to sugars, starches (enriched flour) and saturated fats. These include but are not limited to pastries, candy, white rice, white bread, soda pops, butter, frying oil, cheeseburgers, pizza, etc.

Eliminating these foods will help the body to start expelling the worse of the toxins, and it also will burn 5-7 pounds (*or more*) of body fat per week. I realize that this is not a *'weight-loss'* program per-se. However, you **CAN** expect to lose weight. This is an ancillary benefit if you are overweight. If you already follow a clean diet and/or are not overweight, you may skip this step – although I highly encourage you to restrict your eating before and during the three-phase detox.

If you have read **The 10-Day 'At-Home' Colon Cleansing Formula**, you will note that I recommend a similar diet there. This diet is extremely powerful. It has kept me lean and healthy for many years. And most of the massive cravings that made my life miserable have disappeared. For a complete manual on how to implement this diet as a lifestyle, I invite you to check out The 'Permanent Weight Loss' Diet. Let's take a look at the foods to avoid ...

Banned Foods

*****Salt** - this is something that many of us simply eat too much of. Almost every good that we eat contains sodium. The body receives more than enough without one having to season food with more salt. It was a bit tough for me at first because I was so accustomed to loading most of my foods with it. Food without salt tasted bland and boring. But, you know what? I got used to it. Amazingly, within the first month I also lost 15 pounds, water weight that I was retaining due to abusing salt. I don't miss it at all. I have learned to enjoy the natural taste of food without piling on condiments. Not all seasonings are banned, however. I will get more into that in a little while. But please... if you tend to eat a lot of salt, then I recommend that you cut it out, at the very least until you are done with the detox program.

* **Sugar** – I can safely tell you without exaggeration that sugar was (and is), by far, my number one enemy. It really does absolutely nothing for my body except to induce cravings (for more sugar) and cause me to gain weight. If you are overweight, then you probably know exactly what I'm talking about. Nothing has helped me more over the years to stay lean and healthy than to ban sugar and consume very little of it. At first it was a battle. My entire being wanted sugar, sugar and more sugar. But after a few weeks the cravings went away.

I lost a great deal of body fat, felt more energetic and slept better. My entire health boomed. In short, I implore you to stay away from refined sugar while you are going through this detox. Some fruit like apples, pears and strawberries are fine. These, however, should also be limited.

* **Fried Foods** – Anything fried needs to be eliminated. I'm not saying that you can't use cooking oil at all. You can cook a very nice (and healthy) piece of chicken with just a dab of olive oil, without having to dunk the meat in a pool of grease. Fried foods not only increase bad cholesterol levels, but they also cause obesity and, like sugar, perpetuate cravings that lead to binging and overeating.

* **Cheese** – I am a cheese fanatic. Nonetheless, I have come to respect it because it does (in most cases) have high amounts of fat. I don't know if you have ever tried the so-called 'low-fat' cheese brands, but – in my opinion – they taste absolutely horrible. Mozzarella cheese is the one with the least amount of fat and I do eat in on occasion. Cheddar, Swiss and Gouda cheeses are out for now. Again, you want to

keep the digestive process as light as possible so that the body can focus on detoxification and healing.

* **Dairy Products** - dairy has a lot of fat, is high in sugar content and has been known to cause digestive system inflammation. I myself am lactose intolerant. Anytime that I drink milk, I swiftly bloat like a balloon and explode in terrible flatulence. Sorry, that was probably **TMI** (too much information). But seriously, while you are detoxifying, stay away from whole milk. Drink non-fat instead. Anything above that is banned for now. If you drink whole milk, you are consuming one gram of fat for every ounce. So if you drink an eight-ounce glass of whole milk, you basically just took in eight grams of fat. And you have not even started eating! By simply switching to 2% percent milk, an eight ounce glass of milk goes down from eight to four grams of fat - a pretty dramatic 50 percent reduction!

* **Red Meat** - I personally don't have anything against red meat. In fact, I have been known to eat a piece of meat on rare occasion. Right now, we are banning it because it has a lot of fat, and because,

again, we want to make this entire process as easy as possible for the digestive system. If you eat meat, stick to chicken and fish.

* **Alcohol** - Alcohol is packed with empty calories. Calories with **ZERO** nutritional value. And alcohol turns to sugar. Bad all over. If you drink frequently, cut it down to a minimum. You're doing this for your health and to reach a goal that is important to **YOU**. If you have to go a few days without drinking, your arm is not going to fall off. You'll live. A cup of wine with dinner is fine, but nothing more than that at this juncture.

* **Butter or Margarine** - As they say in New York, "Forget about it!!!" Butter and margarine are pure fat and we don't want it. I realize that this may be blasphemy for some people. How can one eat a piece of toast without butter? That was exactly my sentiment when I first changed my diet. I had to put butter or margarine on everything, even my cereal. Well, not really... but I was a butter/margarine addict. Today, I am happy to eat toast, potatoes and hot cereals (among other foods) without having to pack on the fat. The main problem, especially in the US, is that people eat too much fat. Most have no clue how much fat is in the food they eat. **Quick Note**: One gram of fat is ten calories, and one gram of carbohydrates is four calories. The bottom line is that eating too much fat is what makes people fat. The body only needs twenty to thirty grams of fat per day, yet most obese and overweight people I come across can easily consume more than one hundred grams of fat per day. The rule of thumb is that **you should have no more than 15 grams of fat with each meal.** One pat of butter is ten grams of fat. Some people have a big meal and put one pad on each bread roll they eat and several on their baked potato. If you had two rolls of bread, you can easily be looking at 40 grams of fat just with the bread and potato! And even if it is just one pat for the bread and one for the potato, that is already twenty grams of fat. Enough said.

* **Salad Dressings** - Salad dressing is a huge stumbling block for many people. Many say they are dieting with salads, but fail to realize just how fattening the salad dressing they are using actually is. Salad dressing is made from vegetable oil. Oil, of course, is a

type of fat. So, for example, one ounce (30 ml) of your typical salad dressing has -- on the average -- 15 grams of fat! That is almost enough fat for the whole day in just one ounce of dressing! And I was never satisfied with just one ounce of anything. Many people go to a restaurant and order a large salad as the main meal and pat themselves on the back for not gorging on the wrong type of foods. But then they defeat their efforts by putting two or three ounces of rich dressing on their salads.

At fifteen grams an ounce, that is almost fifty grams of fat - enough for two-and-a-half-days! Salad or no salad, that is still destructive and toxic eating. There are many very good "light" salad dressings you can substitute which will cut your salad fat intake down to roughly two grams of fat per ounce. Now 13 grams less of fat per ounce is a shocking difference, don't you think? I do not recommend the "Fat Free" dressings.

They usually taste funny and will only frustrate you. If you use vinegar and oil in your salad, please know that oil is pure fat - ten grams per ounce. So that also can be a catch 22.

* Fruit Juices - If you read the label of most orange juice brands, you will see that the sugar content is through the roof. Yes, it is natural sugar, but sugar nonetheless. You can have one glass of juice in the morning, but you need to water it down 50/50. Drinking straight juice at this phase is basically like injecting blubber directly into your belly. Stay away. Drink veggie juice instead...but make sure that it is the low sodium veggie juice. :-)

*White Enriched Bread - That stuff is like dropping a ball of cement into the stomach. White flour, doughy garbage really is terrible for human health. I was going to ban all breads, but I remembered that the Ezekiel brand (green bag) is actually very good. You can eat one slice here and there as partial replacement to your carbohydrate servings. We'll get into all of that in just a minute.

*Junk Food of <u>ANY</u> Kind - I think that it definitely goes without saying that junk food is out. And not just out for a little while. Hopefully, it is out of your life for good. That crap is like wearing a ball and chain. It enslaves us to cravings that are never satisfied and only get stronger and more violent. Junk food is like smoking cigarettes. One is to many and one thousand aren't enough.

Foods to Limit:

*Fruit – As already mentioned, stick to apples, pears, strawberries and also cantaloupe. You can also eat an orange occasionally. But citrus are high in acid and we want to make sure not to irritate the digestive system.

* Tomatoes - Tomatoes are also high in acid. If you have eaten poorly for a long time, it is best to limit them so as to minimize digestive system irritation. I am not saying at all that tomatoes are bad. They aren't. Tomatoes are low in sodium and have very little fat or cholesterol. They also are a great source of Niacin, Vitamin B6, Vitamin A, Vitamin C and Vitamin E, among others. We're limiting their consumption simply to minimize acidity and help the digestive system during detoxification.

* Peas or Corn - Peas and corn can be high

in sugar, so please eat them sparingly. I'm not trying to be a sugar cop here. I just want you to get **MAXIMUM** results in these 30 days.

* **Olive Oil** – I already talked about oil above, so I don't want to beat a dead horse. Still, be careful and use olive oil very sparingly at this time.

Ok, now what?

Starting immediately, eliminate **ALL** of these foods and beverages from your diet... period.

This is the beginning of the process. For now, continue to eat whatever else you have been eating **EXCEPT** for the foods that are listed above. I want you to take a full step forward and discontinue eating any and all junk. That's the whole point of our work together, right? To help you achieve measurable improvements in your health.

So cut it all out. Do not eat <u>even a little</u> of them anymore. I mean <u>Nothing</u>, <u>No More</u>, <u>Finito</u>, <u>Nada</u>! You are taking the <u>monumental</u> step of removing **ALL** toxic foods from your diet. I use the word *'monumental'* because, in truth, you are now in the minority. The majority of people **NEVER** confront their eating behaviors as you are now doing. And since you won't be dumping more and more crap into your belly, the detox remedies that I am about to give you will be highly effective.

Chapter 3:
Eat Six Times Daily

Eating smaller meals with greater frequency, totaling six meals per day, is one of the strategies that will help you to receive the most benefit from this program. I would strongly encourage you to observe the banned foods, as well as change your eating structure to one of six smaller meals. This method will <u>accelerate your metabolism</u>, meaning that the body can process and eject toxins faster and with greater efficiency. The metabolism is like a fire. Let me give you an analogy to illustrate. Imagine that you were stranded in a very cold place and need to keep a fire burning to survive the night.

Would you be better off dumping a huge amount of firewood at once, or would the fire burn longer and keep you warmer if you added small amounts of wood frequently? Of course, the answer is the latter.

The more frequently you eat (observing the banned foods list), the better you will feel and the more energy you will have.

Consequently, the metabolism will work evenly and continuously, which results in faster weight loss and elimination of toxins.

Having larger meals with less frequency is like dumping a large amount of wood into the fire. You will get one heck of blaze initially, but it will die out sooner and not provide as much heat (energy) as it would if you added wood more sparingly. This is what causes the monster cravings that keep people trapped in binging and overeating for years.

If you want to disconnect the cravings and succeed in detox cleansing, eat more frequently. Please note: **The diet adjustment doesn't have to be hard**. Six meals per day include breakfast, mid-morning snack, lunch, mid-afternoon snack, dinner and evening snack.

So this is not a *'starvation'* diet by any means; you can still eat generously while also meeting your detoxification goals.

The key is *'quality of food,'* and that's what this diet emphasizes.

To help you see how this works, here is a sample menu from a typical day in my life:

Sample Menu

Breakfast 8:00 AM

1 Cup of Oatmeal with 1 Cup Skim Milk, a Handful of Raisins or Plums
Three Egg Whites mixed with, 3 OZ Ground Turkey
1 Cup of Green Tea with Stevia

Mid-Morning Snack 10AM

1 Apple or Pear Mixed With One Cup of Nonfat Yogurt (Plain) OR, ONE Apple, Pear, Banana or Other Fruit

Lunch - Noon

Big salad with lettuce, tomato and other veggies you may like.
For dressing, use olive oil (no more than 1 teaspoon) and balsamic vinegar.
1 Envelope of Low-Sodium Tuna
1 4OZ Baked Potato or Sweet Potato

Mid-Afternoon Snack 3PM

Same as before - I usually have a piece of fruit mixed with non-fat, plain yogurt. At this time in the afternoon, I also drink another cup of green tea. Green tea has energy-boosting and body-heating properties. It will help to give you a pep as well as calm hunger pangs. In addition to green tea, seltzer water (sparkling water/club soda) is great to navigate hunger.

Dinner - 6PM

Six-to-eight ounces of chicken, fish or ground turkey (I like to make turkey patties)
Large salad as the one eaten for lunch
Steamed Broccoli, Cauliflower and Carrots (most supermarkets have prepackaged vegetable combinations that are ready to steam and eat).
4OZ Baked Potato or Sweet Potato OR 4OZ of Whole Wheat or Whole Grain Pasta OR 4 OZ of Brown Rice

Evening Snack - 8PM

Big salad with 3OZ Chicken, Fish or Ground Turkey - No carbohydrates.
A piece of fruit with Non-fat Yogurt
Cup of Chamomile Tea - Chamomile tea is great to drink at night because it will help soothe hunger as well as calm you and get you ready for bed.

You should not eat anything at least two hours prior to turning in. Sometimes I also take one 500 mg tablet of Tryptophan at night to help me sleep. Tryptophan is an awesome amino acid that helps to stabilize mood.

At this point I'm done eating for the day and drink only water until 8AM the following morning. Again -> **NEVER EAT FOR THE LAST TWO HOURS BEFORE YOU GO TO BED**. Do you ingest a large portion of your daily calories a few hours before bedtime?

When your body is at rest, all of your metabolic processes slow down so you don't burn as many calories as you would during the day while you are actively moving around. When you eat large portions of food shortly before you go to bed, many of those calories are going to be stored as fat. Unfortunately, some people eat very few calories all day long, then gulp down a large dinner – and then munch on snacks all evening before they go to bed!

Throughout the day they may have ingested 500 to 700 calories, and then 2,000 to 3,000 more right before going to bed. Bad idea! Tape your mouth shut if you have to. But eat no more!

Chapter 4:
Detox Symptoms

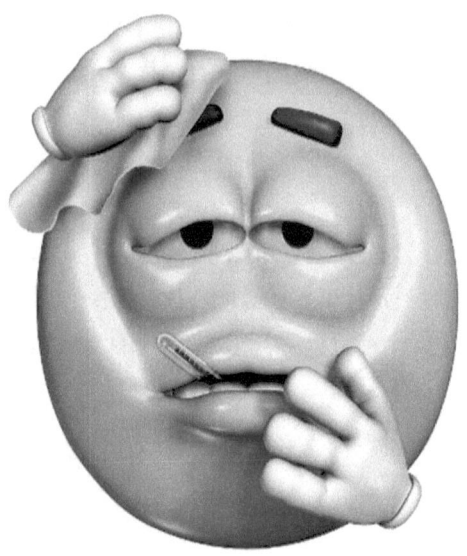

If your diet has been less that optimal, it is likely that adjusting your meals as I've instructed will bring on a variety of symptoms.

As I mentioned earlier, discomfort means that the body is detoxifying, so please do not be discouraged.

Rather, be enthused that your health (and weight) will drastically improve as a result of your efforts. Seriously, the benefits that you stand to gain are really tremendous. Here's a list of the most common 'healing' symptoms:

Headaches – This one is especially marked for coffee drinkers, but is also the case for persons who consume large amounts of sugar and alcohol. This symptom can really take a person out of commission. A lot of my colleagues call me a heretic for saying this, but if you need to take a couple of ibuprofen tablets to ease the pain, then so be it. Usually two tablets will do the trick. But don't take more than four daily. You may need to go through a little pain and discomfort. The good news is that headaches rarely last more than 72 hours, if that.

Dizziness – The body is not used to being deprived of eating whatever it wants and will go through dizzy spells, particularly during the first 11 days. The best solution for dizziness is to move slowly and get as much rest as your daily schedule allows.

Difficulty Performing Basic Tasks – Since you are restricting your food intake, it will take some time for the body to adjust. You may feel very weak and may have trouble getting around - particularly during the first 10-14 days. If you slow down and work on focusing on the individual tasks you are performing, this symptom can be overcome. It is important for you to realize that your body is going through a transition. You must move slowly and not try to push yourself too hard. You may not be able to function at the same capacity as you are accustomed. Fine. Slow down and give the body time to work on your behalf.

Weakness means that you need to be extra careful when walking around, and especially when getting up from a sitting position. Avoid harsh and/or abrupt movements. Move slowly, watch your step closely and always have something that you can hang on to if you suddenly feel like you are fainting. This is good advice. One time I totally hit the deck because I got up to quickly from a chair. I missed the corner of the wall by centimeters, but still hit myself quite hard on the floor. This is about improving our health, not about getting hurt. Please be careful. I mean it. Be careful.

Pulsating Hunger Pains that disappear and then re-emerge throughout the day. For some persons, hunger is monstrous in the morning. But for the vast majority, the hunger troll shows up mostly at night. In short, hunger will always be a part of our lives, and it is our task to master it rather than allow it to enslave us as it **CAN AND WILL** if we let it.

In my case, hunger was very strong in the first week to 10 days of following this diet. Then I found myself getting used to always being 'a little' hungry. After a while, I loved it because I began to feel more alert, more energetic, optimistic... I slept better. I actually **SLEPT THROUGH THE NIGHT** and woke up feeling terrific. Before the diet, I constantly woke up at night to urinate, or like a raving lunatic wanting to raid the fridge. After a while, I would go to sleep at 11PM, close my eyes and, when I opened them, it was 6AM! For me, this was nothing less than a total miracle. And I felt great... refreshed and ready to go! All of that just from getting used to eating less and being a little hungry. Much better than getting stuffed like a boar as I used to.

Bad Breath, Metallic Taste in Mouth, White Sticky Film on Tongue – These are all good indications that your body is eliminating toxicity. Most of these symptoms pass after 14 days (on average). Bad Breath, I suggest that you get sugarless mints and keep them handy until the process ends.

Metallic Taste In the Mouth usually means that there are excessive (and toxic) heavy metals accumulated in your system. I recall having this constant sulfur and 'steel' taste in my mouth for about a week.

White Sticky Film on the Tongue can be disgusting, but it's a sign that the body is cleansing. For these symptoms, the best thing you can do is to keep drinking a lot of water. Make sure to brush your teeth regularly. Keep a travel toothbrush with you if you spend a lot of time out. Mouthwash is also helpful.

Diarrhea or Constipation – All of the fecal matter adhered to your colon will either start gushing out in diarrhea or incite short-term constipation. I know that this is disgusting, but it happens. If you have eaten poorly for a long time, or have simply abused sugar or fat, your body may respond to the cleansing diet by starting to expel all of the toxic filth in this fashion.

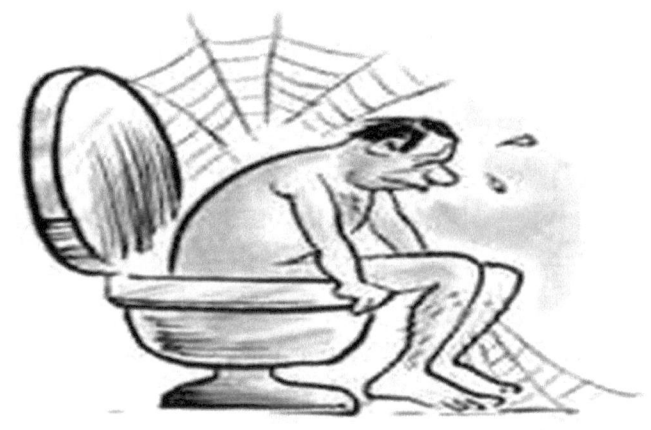

"A common fasting detox symptom is that all of the fecal matter adhered to your colon will either start gushing out in diarrhea or incite short-term constipation. The cobwebs are an exaggeration."

If **Diarrhea** Strikes, simply continue to follow the diet as outlined. Should it become severe, see your pharmacist and ask him or her for an over-the-counter recommendation. Continue with the intermittent fast. Making eating-habit changes is a shock to the body, but it will finally get the message and react favorably to what you are doing. If you have diarrhea, make sure to keep yourself hydrated. **Make it a point to drink at least one gallon of water daily.** Stay close to a bathroom at all times. If you go out, make sure that you are always aware where the nearest restroom is. Seriously, you want to get to the toilet promptly anytime you need to.

If **Constipation** is the case, visit your local pharmacy and ask your pharmacist about a stool softener. I personally use a herbal laxative called Herbs & Prunes. It works like a charm every time and is not harsh on my stomach. Take one tablet to start. Do not exceed four tablets in one day. But do this only if you fail to eliminate anything for at least three days. Give your body enough time to do it on its own.

Irritability / Mood Swings – If you have ever seen The Flintstones, you may remember Fred walking around growling on the episode where he is placed on a diet. Sooooo, be prepared to be a little *"short-*

fused" when you first start this diet. Be aware that you will not be as patient as you normally would. Tell your loved ones not to take it personally if - initially - you are less social that what they are accustomed. This is normal and will pass.

Facial Puffiness & Feeling Bloated – This symptom is much more marked for persons who consume large amounts of salt and/or sugar. I personally was bloated to the max like the Stay Puft Marshmallow man. So being puffy was nothing new. I looked like somebody had stuck huge balloons on my cheeks. It was hideous. The cleansing diet took care of that and my face today is that of a normal human being rather than a cartoon character.

That is a lot of symptoms, but rarely does **ONE** person experience them all. And remember, they will subside and mostly pass after approximately 14 days. Continue to surrender to the process and stay put. Let the body do what it does best. Your body knows how to take care of you. Your body and digestive system thank you for this break. Your body is loyal and noble ... it is unleashing amazing weight loss and healing power even as we speak. All you have to do is hang on and let the process run its course. The kidney, liver and parasite detoxification process has its own individual symptoms which I will discuss within each of those respective chapters. The symptoms listed above (related specifically to the cleansing diet) are temporary. As I said, I've been following this structure for many years and, today, I hardly ever feel any hunger or cravings. So hang in there and give it your very best. You won't regret it! :-)

Note: Of course, if at any time you see that any of these symptoms continue and do not go away (*particularly after 11 days*), then you may have a more serious condition and should visit a medical practitioner at once. It is certainly not my intention to tell you not to see your doctor or to neglect symptoms of what could be a more serious illness.

Chapter 5:
The Kidney Cleanse

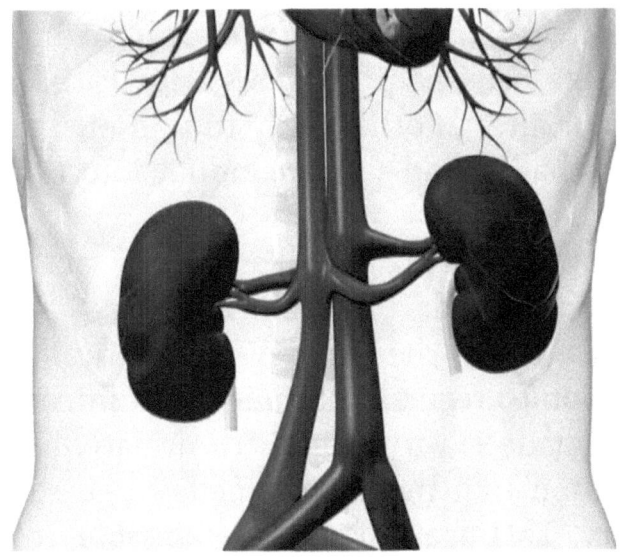

Kidneys are one of the most vital organs in the body. If you have abused your body with poor eating habits, then this kind of cleansing will help to minimize the damage. The kidneys act as filters that remove toxins from the blood stream. They also help to maintain fluid and Electrolyte balance.

In short, the kidneys excrete the liquid waste that accumulates as part of the body's normal metabolic functions. The kidneys are located above the waist on both sides of the spine.

Many people who suffer from chronic lower-back pain would recover via kidney detoxification. A friend of mine suffered terrible back pain for years. He visited one doctor after another, only to find out much later that he had a severe kidney infection.

He swiftly detoxified his kidneys and the pain vanished. I myself have had a few scares with the kidneys, specifically in relation to recurring urinary tract infections that made it very painful to urinate, not to mention that my urine smelled like sulfur. Sorry, **TMI** again! But it was terrible, to say the least. It was following the kidney cleansing formula presented here that my infections went away for good – and so did that awful smell.

Kidney Conditions

When the kidneys are not functioning properly, metabolic waste begins to build up in the body. This retention can cause a condition called <u>Uremia</u>, which, if not treated, can result in life-threatening <u>Renal Failure</u>. Waste retention is also related to other toxic conditions such as Gout. Very widespread in our culture are Kidney Stones – toughened mineral deposits that can be **VERY** painful. If not passed, kidney stones can block the flow of urine and cause a recurring and severe Urinary Tract Infection, as was the case with me. A cleanse will wash out the kidneys so that stones can be passed easily. It also assists in the satisfactory formation and passageway of urine. The links above will take you to Wikipedia for more information on each of the named conditions.

Chapter 6:
Kidney Detox Remedy

Here are the items that you will need to prepare the kidney detox remedy:

Organic Apple Juice - Apple juice helps the body fight-off bad cholesterol while enhancing cardiovascular health. It also combats constipation, cleans the liver and kidneys and is known to boost intestinal/colon health.

Gravel Root Tablets - Herbal support for kidneys and gallbladder. Supports normal detoxification processes. Features gravel root, parsley root and marshmallow root, historically used to promote healthy elimination of fluids from the kidneys. Includes the bitter herbs dandelion root and turmeric, to support the normal flow of bile from the gallbladder.

BearBerry-Uva Ursi - Promotes urinary tract health.

Parsley 450mg Capsules – Antioxidant, anti-cancer, anti-inflammatory.

Hydrangea Root Tincture - Diuretic to help soothe mucous membranes or urinary tract.

Further along, you also will need:

Magnesium Oxide 400mg

Vitamin B6 100mg

Average Cost for This Remedy-> $65

Chapter 7:
Kidney Cleanse Directions

Do this cleanse for **FIVE** days. In an 8-to-12-ounce coffee cup or mug, mix:

• 8 Ounces of Organic Apple Juice
• 20-30 Drops of Hydrangea Root Tincture
• 20-30 Drops Uva Ursi

Prepare the remedy in the morning (before breakfast) and drink it at once. The taste can be slightly bitter. Follow it up with a 12-ounce glass of water. When you are finished, have your breakfast as usual. After eating, take:

(1) Capsule Ginger Root
(1) Capsule Parsley AND
(1) Capsule Gravel Root.

At the end of the five days, discontinue the above and begin taking **ONE Cap of Vitamin B6** and **Magnesium Oxide** DAILY to help maintain kidney health. Rest for 24-48 hours before proceeding to the Phase 2 Parasite Elimination remedy. Very Important:

Please make sure to drink at least half-a-gallon of water every day.

Kidney Cleanse Side Effects

*Feeling anxious and/or irritable: You may feel very restless and unable to relax. If that is the case, drink Chamomile tea and, at night, if insomnia strikes, one (or two at most) tablet of Tryptophan can help you sleep.

*An acidic, foul smell over the body, especially the arms and arm-pits. I recommend that you use plenty of deodorant if you have to be around others (or even for yourself!). When you bathe, thoroughly scrub your skin to ensure that the released toxins (or any lingering inside the pores) are washed away.

*Sulfuric/metallic scent when urinating, indicating the release of excess uric acid. As I mentioned earlier, I went through several days where the smell of my urine was simply unbearable. But remember: these symptoms are a sign that the detox is working and that you are going to emerge healthier and stronger than before. :-)

*Weakness, sadness (emotionalism): This symptom is not very common, but it may surface. If so, just be good to yourself and realize that it is all part of the detox process. The emotional upheaval will level out in the proceeding days. If you find yourself struggling with extreme mood swings, you can take a <u>magnesium tablet</u> to help stabilize (you can use the same magnesium oxide indicated in the remedy). It is recommended that you get as much rest as possible during any detox cleanse. Give your body the energy and time it needs to do the miracle on your behalf! I like to take warm/hot water baths, which are very relaxing and also stimulate the further release of toxins.

*Pain from the passing of stones. If you have kidney stones, you may have pain which can be from mild to severe. In most cases, however, the discomfort will be minimal. Make sure to follow the remedy preparation instructions to the letter and you'll be on your way.

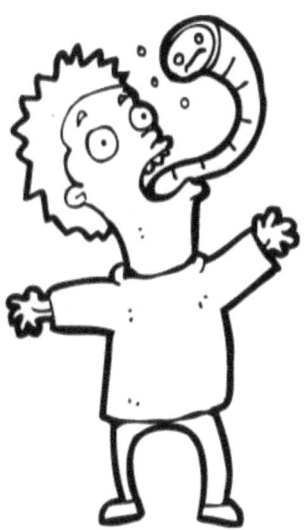

"Parasites take advantage of our body's weakness and can, in some cases, hasten the development of chronic illness."

Chapter 8: Parasite Detoxification

I don't know about you, but just saying the word "parasites" makes me grimace. These invaders take advantage of our body's weakness and can, in some cases, hasten the development of chronic illness. If you have been overweight for a long time and your diet is filled with junk, then this cleanse is definitely for you.

Why? Because, **through poor eating and obesity, the digestive system becomes clogged and creates the perfect living environment for parasites.** So, while this topic can be quite gross, it is nonetheless a crucial part of our training as we endeavor to improve our health for the **LONG TERM.**

I don't want to scare you, but parasite infection is more common than one may think. Estimates from various international medical authorities indicate that more than 70% of the world's population is host to parasite infection.

Parasites cause some of the **Worst Diseases** on our planet. Malaria alone affects millions of people every year, many cases resulting in death.

What is a Parasite?

A parasite is basically an organism that feeds on and/or lives inside another, such as an animal or human body. It can live in your digestive system, organs and even the blood. Parasites include different types of worms, insects, protozoan and other microscopic organisms which feed on the host but do not contribute to its survival.

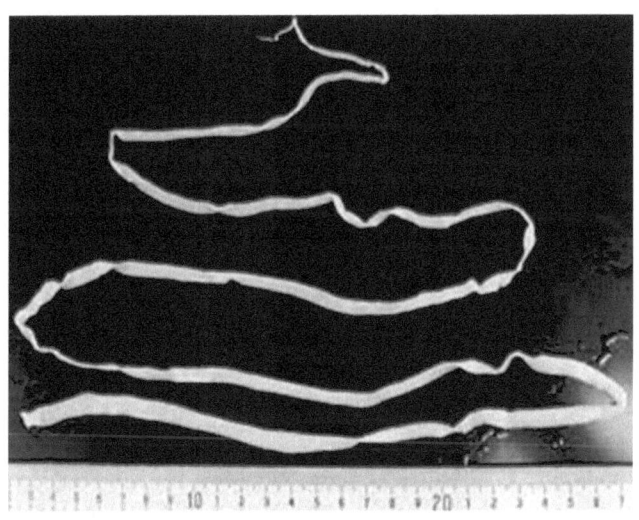

Parasites will vary in size from one-thousandth of a micron to the whale tapeworms (pictured above) which can grow as long as 120 feet. The longest recorded tapeworm pulled out of a human was **37 feet long**. Parasite "types" that we are vulnerable to include: <u>Ascaris</u>, <u>Hookworms</u>, <u>Whipworms</u>, <u>Pinworm</u>, (*most common in children*), <u>Giardia</u> and <u>Trichina Worms</u> which cause the disease <u>Trichinosis</u>.

Years ago I lived in Central America and was stricken with a horrible parasite infestation that nearly killed me. I was horribly sick for weeks. Anytime I went to the bathroom – which was constantly – I could see some of these parasites *"swimming around"* in the water before I flushed. **DEFINITELY** too much information! Sorry. I just want to emphasize that this is definitely for real. Now that is an extreme case. But believe me, these suckers are mean and vicious. Furthermore, whether you are mildly or severely contaminated, the remedy that I am about to give you will wipe them out. I want you to keep your focus, not on the discomfort or grossness, but rather on the huge health improvements that you are going to receive.

That state of mind is the one that keeps me going when challenges arise.

How Does One Get Parasites?

A common way to get infected with parasites is through pets. If you have a dog, cat or even a bird, then you are susceptible every time you pet, bathe and/or brush them **AND** when they peck or lick you. It is for this reason that doctors usually tell pregnant women **NOT** to clean cat litter boxes or be "*too close*" to pets. A good practice is to always wash your hands after grooming animals.

I have three cats and clean three litter boxes daily. Yes, these cats are spoiled and each one insists on having its own private box. What can I tell you? They rule the house! At any rate, always wear gloves when cleaning poop, whether it be cats, birds, dogs or exotic reptiles. I use disposable rubber gloves. When I'm done I throw them out (of course), wash my hands in hot water and apply disinfectant.

In recent years, awareness related to having clean hands has surged. And rightfully so!

We touch a myriad of different things throughout the day. We don't know who touched them before or if they were healthy or not. So, indeed, wash your hands regularly throughout the day. Keep a small bottle of disinfectant with you. Today, when one walks into a supermarket, it is not uncommon to see wipes at the entrance. By all means use them.

Moreover, parasite infestation can happen via the consumption of improperly prepared foods. This includes undercooked meat, poultry, or fish. It can also be caused by not correctly washing fresh vegetables and fruits. I'm 99.9% certain that the terrible bout I had with parasites was caused by meat that was not properly cooked. Another important tip I can give you is this: Never cut produce on the same surface used for raw meat. If you cut meat on your counter or on a cutting board, make sure to wash the surface thoroughly with hot water and soap before you lay veggies on it (*or any other kind of food*).

Water (even chlorinated tap water) can also harbor parasites. No matter where you live, I strongly encourage you to invest in a good water filter; avoid tap water. Or at the very least, boil the water for five minutes before drinking (*wait for it to cool before you do of course!*). In addition, parasites can enter the body through wet grass and/or standing water. Abstain from walking barefoot outside as much as possible. I am not saying that you should become paranoid about getting parasites. Instead, I want you to exercise preventive caution, plain and simple.

Do I Have Parasites?

There are actual laboratory tests to establish whether or not one has parasites. However, most of those tests only detect 30 to 40 different types. It is therefore **<u>VERY</u>** possible for one to test negative and still have parasites.

Of course, there are many different symptoms of a parasite infestation. Why? Because they don't just infect one part of the body. Also, some are only detectable during certain life cycles. To be sure, parasites are one of the primary causes for diseases and can greatly harm the immune system.

They are regularly missed during the diagnosis of many chronic health problems. Parasites can truly be *"The Quiet Killer"*.

Hopefully, in years to come, their recognition can **<u>FINALLY</u>** assist the medical community to solve the enigma surrounding many diseases. Here are a few parts of the body where parasites lurk, and the related symptoms:

Lymphatic System: Allergies could be a symptom of parasites in the Lymphatic System, particularly as digested food goes to the intestines.

A lot of parasites move in and out of the lymphatic system, which can often be overlooked or diagnosed as something else. Tropical *"parasite-based"* diseases as Filariasis are becoming more and more common.

Joints or Tissue: Inflamed arthritis or other muscle/joint pain may be a sign of parasites. They can form cysts and create inflammations; the resulting pain often attributed to arthritis.

Mucous Membrane: Problems with the bladder, lungs, sinuses, or vagina, for example, may be worsened by the presence of a parasite.

The Digestive System: Manifests in something as plain as indigestion, constipation, as well as other types of tenderness in the stomach, Colitis, or even ulcers. Puncture of the intestinal walls by parasites causes big amounts of undigested molecules to go into the abdominal cavity which can produce in infections such as Peritonitis.

Skin: Itching, swelling, rashes, and even psoriasis, eczema and hives are possible signs of a parasitic contagion.

In general: Fatigue (especially after eating) and Anemia may be indicative of parasites in the body. Parasites can even travel into the brain. They can form Granulomas in the lungs, liver, uterus or other organs. Parasites' toxic metabolic products attack the central nervous system causing restlessness, depression, anxiety and hypertension.

Now let me repeat: it is certainly **NOT** my intention to advocate that we become "parasite paranoid" ... seeing parasites everywhere and being scared to drink water or walk on the grass barefoot. We must enjoy life. But we **CAN** do what is within our reach to protect ourselves in reasonable ways, right? That **IS** what this program is all about!

Chapter 9:
Parasite Remedy

Here are the items required to prepare the parasite remedy:

Apple Juice (Organic) – As we saw above in the kidney detox chapter, Apple juice helps the body fight-off bad cholesterol while enhancing cardiovascular health. It also combats constipation, cleans the liver and kidneys and is known to boost intestinal/colon health.

L-ornithine 500mg - You will also need it for the liver detox remedy. Various studies have shown that ornithine can help boost energy and counteract fatigue/weakness, reduce stress and fight cirrhosis (liver disease). Ornithine is also used by many athletes and weight lifters to increase HGH (human growth hormone) levels.

Wormwood Combination - Wormwood is the sour herb that gives vermouth its distinct taste. For our purposes, we will use wormwood to repel any and all parasites that may be hiding/afflicting your body, particularly the digestive system. It seems that parasites do not like the smell of wormwood and, once ingested, they start to jump ship through bowel movements. I know that this sounds extremely disgusting, and I want you to prepare yourself to (*possibly*) see parasites in your toilet bowl during this process. Just be grateful that those suckers are **OUT** of your body. God riddance, I say... so please don't be alarmed. Interestingly, wormwood is said to increase a person's psychic abilities and, if burned at a cemetery, can summon the spirit of the dead. In our case, however, it is **DEAD** parasites that we're after, and wormwood will certainly deliver! :-)

Black Walnut Hull Tincture – black walnut is anti-bacterial, fungicidal, and anti-parasitic. Tannins are polyphenols thought to help resist many conditions such as blood disorders, stress, tumors, ulcers and cancer. Iodine, required by most living creatures, has been widely used as an antiseptic. Additionally, black walnut tinctures have been used to treat bilious conditions and cramp colic.

Clove Capsules 500mg – Clove is used to treat nausea and relieve pain. It also helps to kill intestinal parasites and treat fungal and bacterial infections as well as digestive system disturbances.

Probiotics – Basically, probiotics are 'good' bacteria that assist digestion and help maintain digestive system health. Our digestive system has hundreds of these helpful bacteria, which are essential to fight off the 'bad' ones. Probiotic bacteria are comprised mostly of yeast and lactic acid or Lactobacillus acidophilus, found in yogurt.

Average Cost for This Remedy-> $45

Chapter 10:
Parasite Killer Instructions

Now that I have scared the bejesus out of you, let's move forward with the solution to this parasite dilemma.

Do This:

• If possible, start the parasite detox when the moon is full. That is when parasites are known to be most active.

• Take the herbal combination described below at least **45 minutes prior to three meals**. Make sure you do it on an empty stomach.

• At night, take as many as four L-ornithine capsules if you find that you cannot sleep.

Week 1: Add 30 drops of the black walnut hull to one cup of organic apple juice. Drink the mixture with one capsule of wormwood and one capsule of cloves.

Take this dosage 3 times daily.

The best times of the day are: in the morning upon awakening, one hour before lunch and one hour prior to eating dinner.

Week 2: Continue with 30 drops of black walnut hull and one cup of the apple juice. However, Increase the wormwood and cloves to 2 capsules each. Take this mixture three times per day as indicated above.

Week 3: Stay at 30 drops of the black walnut hull to one cup of organic apple juice. Increase the wormwood and cloves to 3 capsules each. Take this dose of herbs 3 times per day as already indicated.

The majority of parasites will die over the first 7 days, but keep going for at least **THREE WEEKS** (and as long as three months). Some people decide to keep going for three months to ensure total cleansing. If you decide to go past three weeks, do so with the **SAME DOSAGE** from week three.

DO NOT, in your zeal for getting well, exceed the dosages specified above. Follow the amounts exactly as they were given. This detox can be done in combination with the others. And, of course, stick to the diet that we talked about as closely as possible. The leaner your diet is while you are doing this detox, the better (*and faster*) will be the results.

Final Words

Remember to drink plenty of water each day to accelerate the flush-out of toxins. Parasites are prevalent in a lot of our environment, so I would recommend that you repeat this detox annually. Children are particularly vulnerable to parasites because everything they see usually ends up in their mouths. Teenagers can take adult dosages.

Please consult a Holistic/Alternative Medicine Doctor for dosages if you suspect your child has parasites. Although there aren't any specific symptoms related to a parasite cleanse, you **MAY** experience a Healing Crisis. This "crisis" is usually comprised of headaches, fever, dizziness, diarrhea and an overall "flu-like" feeling. Most people feel nothing, but some with more severe parasite infections **DO** experience symptoms. The key word I want to emphasize is "healing".

Whatever you feel physically, keep in mind it is happening because your body is ridding itself of these dangerous pests. You are getting stronger and healthier! Finally, because of the importance of what we are discussing, let me again run through some practices that will help prevent parasitic infection.

* Wash your hands frequently as they are the primary source of parasite contamination and other infections. Instruct your children to do the same.

* As much as possible, keep your hands away from your mouth, nose, and eyes.

* If you have central air-conditioning, make sure to change the filter at least once per month. There are some premium filters that last as long as three months. You can usually find them at your local supermarket for about $20. If your budget allows it, purchase an air purifier. I got one this past year and was disgusted when I went to clean the filter and saw black spots of filth adhered to it on every side. You mean I was breathing all of that?

* Clean fruits and vegetables **WELL** before eating, especially organically-grown products. As mentioned above, **NEVER** use the same plate or cutting board for salads and vegetables that you do for raw meat.

* Rinse-off meat (steak, chicken, fish) before preparation and cook it thoroughly. Nowadays it is better to cook meat just a little more than you like it to be on the safe side.

* Drink only properly filtered water. I realize that this may sound a tad excessive and, to be fair, most tap water – at least in the US – is drinkable. But I don't want you to settle for just 'drinkable.' I want you to strive for the very highest quality available. If you can, my **TOP** recommendation is that you invest in a water ionizer. Ionized water is, by far, the very best that I've ever tasted.

* Eat yogurt frequently. This helps replenish normal intestinal bacteria, as we already talked about earlier.

* Keep your pets clean and free of parasites. In fact, adult dogs and cats can be given the above remedy also.

*Dispose of pet wastes immediately and wear gloves (*and mask if desired*) when doing so.

* If your immune system is challenged or impaired, take vitamin and mineral supplements. It may be tempting to purchase the less expensive generic versions found in grocery and drug stores, but natural supplements like those in health food stores are of much higher quality. That means that they are absorbed better by the body.

Liver, Gallbladder, Pancreas and Bile Passage

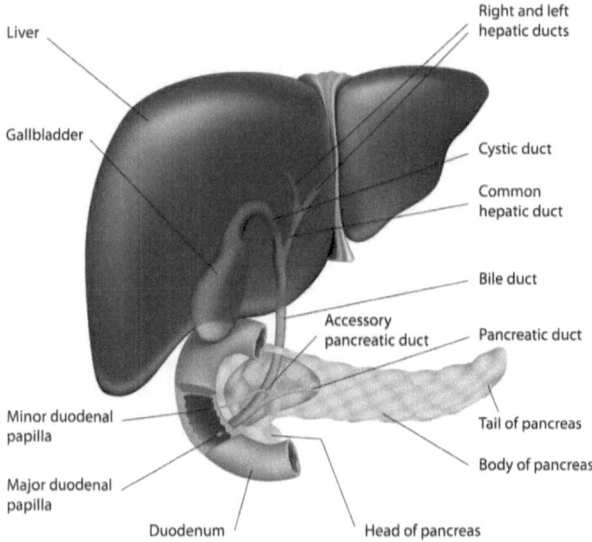

"With proper nutrition and detoxification, even a tired and ill liver can regenerate itself."

Chapter 11:
The Liver Cleanse

The liver is an amazing organ. It is so powerful and loyal that even if you cut out a chunk it will grow back and keep working. With proper nutrition and detoxification, even a tired and ill liver can regenerate itself. This is imperative since the organ is the site of many key metabolic functions. I was challenged with a severe liver condition for many years.

Today, although still present, this illness has virtually no effect on my health. But I have had to do a lot of work via intermittent juice fasting, water fasting **AND** cleanses like the ones we're doing here. The hardest part was quitting cigarettes, which pour hundreds of toxic chemicals into the body. I had to become willing to go to any lengths to achieve my goal.

Signs of Liver Toxicity

Some signs that the liver may be in distress include: poor digestion, abnormal cholesterol levels, recurrent allergies, fatty cysts, cirrhosis, cancer, gallstones and hepatitis. Even if you do **NOT** have liver problems, there are still many benefits to doing this cleanse. Remember: the liver is the primary organ responsible for ridding the body of toxins. This means that everything that we eat, drink and breathe has to be processed by the liver.

The liver manufactures cholesterol and amino acids. It also aids in digestion by taking out surplus glucose, converting it to glycogen, and storing it for energy. The liver removes ammonia – a toxin produced by protein digestion- and turns it into urea so that it can be excreted by the kidneys. The liver secretes bile – *a component needed to digest fat* – and stores it in the gall bladder. For this reason, a good liver cleanse can give your body a tremendous boost in its capacity to process fat.

Before The Liver Cleanse

To undertake this assignment, you will have to plan to fast from one afternoon to the next morning (*approximately 18 hours*). You will also have to be near a bathroom and have ready access to lots of good water.

IMPORTANT: During a cleanse, the liver can excrete notable amounts of toxins into the blood stream. These toxins have to be filtered by the kidneys, which need to be working efficiently to handle the load.

That is why I am putting this liver detox at the end of the program. When you start this, you should have already completed the kidney detox so that your body's filtering system will be fresh and renewed.

The colon will also play a key role in ridding the body of these liver toxins. Therefore, I suggest that you do a colon clean as well before launching the liver detox. I put together a very simple and powerful system to do this on Volume 1- **The 10-Day 'At Home' Colon Cleansing Formula.**

Moreover, it is best if women wait until **AFTER** their menstrual period to do a liver cleanse. As I said, you will need an entire afternoon and the following morning to successfully complete this detox. So do **NOT** do it if you are in a hurry. Make sure that you can spend the time needed to do it thoroughly and without interruptions.

Chapter 12:
Liver Detox Remedy

Ok, we're coming in for the landing. Here are the items that you will need to put together the liver detox remedy:

Extra Virgin Olive Oil - Studies indicate that EVOO could help prevent colon cancer. Extra-virgin olive oil can protect the liver from oxidative stress (cellular damage).

Fresh Grapefruit – Various nutritional studies over the past decade have shown that regular consumption of grapefruit can help prevent liver disease. People with various liver conditions, such as fatty liver, are encouraged to eat grapefruit regularly as part of their treatment. I know that I said earlier that you should eat citrus sparingly. But it is fine to consume it in this case, as long as you do it as indicated.

L-ornithine 500mg – We already looked at this earlier, but here it is again: Ornithine is an amino acid that is involved in the urea cycle, helping to support good liver function, detoxification, and promoting the discharge of growth hormones that break down body fat. Ornithine is believed to enhance the body's immune reaction to bacteria, viruses, and tumors. There is some evidence that Ornithine can also help to treat liver cirrhosis and even improve the performance of athletes, particularly as it relates to muscle growth, body shape and physical strength and endurance.

Epsom Salt – Fosters liver detoxification, boosts liver function and can help relieve constipation.

Milk Thistle 1,000mg - Milk Thistle is an amazing herb (active ingredient is called silymarin) with extremely powerful liver-protecting properties. Having struggled with a liver illness for many years, I know firsthand just how beneficial milk thistle is to help the liver detox, strengthen and heal. In cases of extreme liver poisoning, as in the consumption of the deadly Amanita mushroom, milk thistle is the only treatment option available.

Average Cost for This Remedy-> $40

Chapter 13:
Liver Cleanse Directions

• On the first day of the liver cleanse, stay away from fatty foods. In fact, eat as little as you can, preferably nothing at all.

If you have been following the diet as outlined, you will be in an optimum position to benefit from this remedy.

• Eat your last meal by 3pm the day that you plan on carrying out the procedure.

• At 6pm, drink 3/4 cup of water with **ONE TABLESPOON** of Epsom salt.

• At 8pm of that day, drink another 3/4 cup of water with **ONE TABLESPOON** of Epsom salt.

• At 10pm, drink a mixture of 1/2 a cup of olive oil **AND** the juice from one grapefruit (approx. 3/4 cups of juice). Take **FOUR** L-ornithine capsules and go at once to bed. If you find that you cannot fall asleep, take as many as **FOUR** more L-ornithine caps.

• After 6am the next morning, drink 3/4 cup of water with **ONE TABLESPOON** of Epsom salt.

•Two hours later, drink another 3/4 cup of water with **ONE TABLESPOON** of Epsom salt.

•You may eat a light breakfast after 10am of that day. Eat light meals without too much meat for the rest of the day.

IMPORTANT! The human liver does most of its work during the early AM hours while the body is asleep. Since a lot of other functions are reduced when we are sleeping, this appears to be the best time for the liver to process what we have eaten. It is therefore indispensable that you take the olive oil-grapefruit mixture no later than 10pm. We want to stimulate the liver, but we also want you to have enough time to go to sleep. If you **DO NOT** take the L-ornithine, then you may be in for a very rough night – **WIDE AWAKE!** The water and Epsom salt mixture will induce your body to expel all of the contents in your digestive system. What that means is this: You are going to experience diarrhea.

Make sure to drink lots of water so your body does not dehydrate. The body will need plenty of liquids so it can flush out all of the poisons and toxins accumulated in your liver. In the morning, your bowel movement will likely contain some greenish fatty looking particles ranging anywhere in size from a bean to a lime.

Do not be horrified! Rather, be thankful that your body is getting rid of this garbage. These are toxic deposits that can cause severe illness later on. Begin taking 1,000 mg Milk Thistle daily for a minimum of six months after completing this liver detox.

Once you have finished the liver cleanse, it is time to do a:

Warm Water Enema. Some people are "anti-enema" and run for the door at the slightest mention of "anal insertion". I am confident that you **ARE NOT** one of these people, right? If you **ARE** squeamish, go ahead and do it anyway! Doing a warm water enema **AFTER** a liver detox is **VERY IMPORTANT**. Why? Because it will make sure that **ALL** residual toxins and fatty debris are flushed out of the colon!

You don't want this to be reabsorbed into your body. You have done a lot of cleansing work. Keep moving forward. Do the enema!

It will be important to do this cleanse again in about **TWO** months. Some, more stubborn toxins may remain. A second flush will give them another aggressive push – **OUT!** In some instances, the follow-up cleanse is more dramatic than the first. So please repeat this liver cleanse in roughly eight weeks.

Chapter 14:
Mastering Food

If you have followed my instructions that means that you have done a LOT of work. You have modified your diet, lost weight and thoroughly detoxified your liver and kidneys, and you have wiped out any intestinal parasites that were present. You will have to be careful when you resume your regular diet. The tendency may be to eat in excess as hunger will likely strike very strongly.

If possible, I would recommend that you stick to this diet as closely as possible and learn to navigate hunger and the urge to eat in excess. As a matter of fact, the less you eat after you complete this program, the better you will feel and the more remarkable the results will be. It's all about what we eat, really.

Eating poorly (*or too much*) is what causes our organs to ail. The point we always emphasize is this; permanent weight loss and health are best attained when one is constantly learning about the food one eats, what it contains, and how it positively or negatively is affecting our minds and bodies.

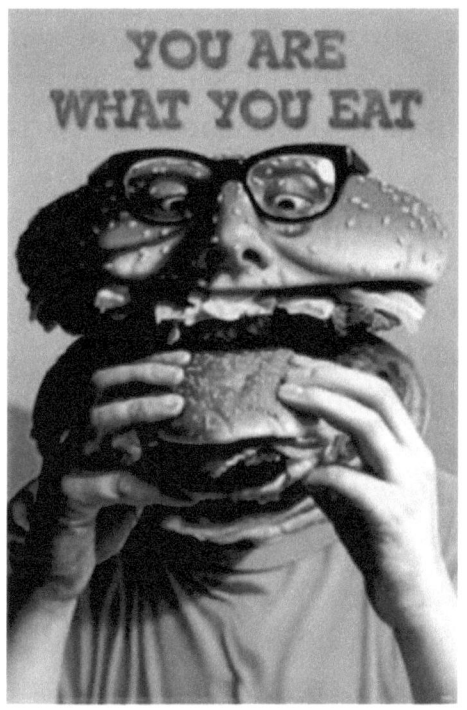

I swam in a pool of ignorance for years; eating whatever and whenever without any clue as to what food was, and how it could help enhance or destroy life. Truly, the picture above is a very good depiction of what I was rapidly becoming through my obesity, binging and overeating. So let us join together in this quest for understanding and, eventually, mastering food. To master food is to master our bodies.

And to master our bodies is to master our minds and emotions. To master our minds and emotions is to master our lives. Believe it or not, your body detox and weight loss quest has existential significance. If you stick to it and resist the urge to return to old habits, I can tell you that the physical and mental breakthroughs that await you are beyond imagination. Food is the source of power - it is up to you to learn how to use it in your favor, rather than as an agent of self-annihilation.

You Are What You Eat

The old adage "You are what you eat," is true. Food can be toxic. The junk food that so many eat in high quantities (*soda, burgers, French fries, pizza, candy etc*) is full of all types of destructive elements that cut many lives short. You probably have heard of many of them, including chemicals, free radicals, as well as excessive amounts of sugar and trans fats. These foods, as we all know, are very high in calories and have little or no nutritional value.

Worse yet, for many people - especially in the US - this type of poisonous food represents the bulk of their daily diets. It is little wonder why the obesity epidemic is spiraling out of control.

Understanding Food

The weight loss and fitness we seek is attained by eating less, of course. But more importantly it is about **eating right**. You can do dozens of liver, colon, kidney and parasite detox programs. However, if you do not take hold of your eating habits, the benefits will be paltry and you will find yourself constantly returning to substandard health. I want you to use food to your advantage rather than to your detriment. One of the most constructive ways you can start using food to your advantage is to **learn how to scrutinize and understand food labels**. This may sound silly, but I have learned that 90 percent of people hardly ever - or never - read labels.

Or perhaps they misread the label, which can be even worse. In the US, the Food and Drug Administration requires that anything in a container (*and almost anything edible you buy*) has to have a label with nutritional facts, including serving size, servings per container, calories, fat, carbohydrates and proteins. We have all seen them, right? Many labels also have in-depth information as to how much sugar and/or salt the particular food contains. As I've already mentioned, I am shocked by the obscene amount of sodium (*salt*) in most canned and frozen foods. This is the case with even so called "diet" or "low fat" selections. When I started to actually read and understand labels, I found that almost 100 percent of what I was eating was toxic and damaging to my body.

Serving Sizes

Please be aware that if the label says that it has "*two servings per container,*" then all the nutritional information in the label of that particular product needs to be doubled. I am sure that you probably know this already, but I think it was worth mentioning for the sake of what we are discussing.

A large container of frozen food may say, for example, "four servings in a box." If you eat the whole box, you are eating four times the amount of fat or calories in the label. In this case the *"serving size"* would be one-fourth of that particular box, not the entire box as many people often believe. Bottom Line, make sure you check both Serving Size and Servings per container. Nine times out of ten the servings per container exceed the serving size, meaning that if you consume that entire product, the fat, calories, carbohydrates etc have to be multiplied times the servings per container.

Chapter 15:
More on Fat, Sugar & Starches

The abuse of fat, sugar and starches and how this practice is literally making millions sick and sending them to an early grave. When you combine this with chronic inactivity, the result undoubtedly is obesity and sickness. It is my aim to give you a message that goes **BEYOND DETOX** so that you can permanently attain a leaner and healthier you. Perhaps starch and inactivity have been a trap for you.

Don't worry. There is a way out. Here we are going to get slightly technical in regards to white starches and sugars and how they negatively affect your body. We also will provide suggestions you can use to get your back on track and help you achieve your weight loss and fitness goals. But as with everything, this is a process. Be good to yourself and remember: the tortoise won the race. Make slow but steady changes and you will definitely reap the results. The fact that you are reading this book already shows that you are motivated to take action. What I want you to do now is to **CONTINUE** to take action until you develop new eating and lifestyle habits that support and enhance the health benefits gained through detoxification.

Starch Sabotage

The other thing you can do is to take a food inventory and remove as much refined starches and sugars from your diet as you can. This time, however, you won't be doing it for only 30 days to do a detoxification program. I want you to do it for good! There is good reason to do this. In the US, there are more stomach diseases than in any other country in the world. The reason? Abuse of starches and sugars - to a great extent. In Asian countries, for the most part, they do not have problems with obesity or the barrage of gastrointestinal problems we see in the West. Stomach cancer, diverticulitis, colitis - all of these diseases are rare. One of my very good friends has been a nurse for more than 30 years and she says she has **NEVER** come across and Asian patient needing a gastric bypass surgery. Maybe one or two have been overweight. Most are lean, she said. During the 16 days I spent in China some years ago, the only overweight people I saw were present only in the large cities of Hong Kong and Beijing. Guess what? That is where the fast food restaurants are! Coincidence? I don't think so. They just do not eat the same way as in the west.

Food Combinations

Thirty years ago, the concept of food combinations came up for the first time. It centers on the premise that, for example, starch and protein should not be eaten together. Refined starches such as bread or potatoes should be eaten with a salad or a vegetable - not meat as it is done customarily.

Why? Because the combination of refined starch and meat often end up becoming an indigestible lump in your stomach. This puts significant strain in your digestive system. In the US, the combination of fat and starch represents the main staple of the diet. What is a hamburger? Fat from the meat, starch from the bread. What is pizza? Fat from the cheese, starch from the dough.

What is a hot dog? What is a submarine sandwich? Same fat/starch combination with a different disguise.

Escaping the Starch and Fat Trap

What is your diet mostly made up of? How do you combine foods and which are the ones that make up the largest portion of your daily consumption? For many overweight (and highly toxic) people, it is almost certain that **fat and starch are combined in almost every meal**. This is a very harmful practice that, over years, can seriously affect your health and cut your life short. I want you to consider removing all "white" starches from your diet or, at the very least, only eat them once a day.

Foods like white rice, white bread, enriched pasta, most breakfast cereals, crackers cookies, cakes and chips, should be seriously curtailed or - better yet - **eradicated**. And remember: fasting even once a week can be a very powerful practice toward weight loss and better health. Or, at the least, try skipping one meal every three days. Do what you can. But do it! It works, it really does!

Chapter 16:
Inactivity

The weight gain/ weight loss equation remains the same: **Calories In - Calories Burned = Weight Loss or Weight Gain**, depending on the amount of calories consumed. We all know that the most successful method to lose weight is attain optimum health is to not only decrease calorie intake, but to also increase the amount of calories burned via some sort of exercise.

I come from a family of mostly heavy people. The genetic predisposition to obesity has been verified along with many other diseases. But this does not mean that you should simply surrender to the fact that you will be obese because other persons from your family are overweight. This is not true. In fact, my message to you is that you **CAN** make the change! You **CAN** break patterns that perhaps other people in your family were unable to overcome.

Upon pondering this thought, I realize that it has been increased physical activity which has helped me the most to stay lean and healthy. I regularly practice the detoxification program that is outlined in this book. However, I am not sure if I would have been able to maintain my health and weight if I wasn't active.

When, for one reason or another, I become inactive, I feel the pain almost immediately. Overall, I always become restless and uncomfortable when I go more than a week without exercising. The insidious thoughts of eating in excess start to circle around my head like vultures.

To me, inactivity is poison. It traps me and causes bad eating habits to reemerge. **And here's the truth:** all living things move - plants, animals, humans. The only organism that is perfectly still is one that is dead.

Why then do beings created to move (*equipped with muscles, ligaments and bones that support and conduce movement*) by their very purpose and design, lie still for days, weeks, months and years? It does not make sense.

Get Moving

When a flower stops blowing in the wind and swaying with the breeze, it is usually laying brown, brittle and dead on the ground. So what can you do? Don't go jogging! Start out with something simple that will not place too much pressure on your joints. Start small like, for example, taking the stairs instead of the elevator when going into a building. Walk around the block twice a week.

Go to the mall and do some window shopping. Walk from one side of the complex to the other. Wherever you go, make it a point to park at a distance and walk. Go to your local video store and rent a low impact beginners exercise tape you can start doing several times a week. Mainly, find something that you enjoy doing. Are you inclined to practice a particular sport? Tai Chi is an excellent form of martial art that is low impact but definitely works you out. What about yoga? Or joining a gym?

The options are truly endless. But you are the one that has to make the commitment to do it. Procrastination is a real killer of dreams and goals. But, be warned: whatever you choose to do as an activity has to be enjoyable. If it becomes a chore, you are not likely to stick to it. I would suggest you draft a list of activities you enjoy taking part of, and make it a point to do them as often as possible. These simple changes in diet and lifestyle will go a LONG way to keep you lean and healthy, making the body detoxification program you learned here much more powerful, effective and beneficial for the long-term.

Chapter 17:
Assignments

1. **Purchase ALL of the Ingredients Needed to Complete the Entire 30-day Detox Program.** Take this book with you to the health food store and make sure that you have everything that you need to complete the entire detox program. t will be much more beneficial to have all of the ingredients handy, so you can focus on the daily preparation and consumption, NOT on having to go out shopping because you forgot or did not get an ingredient. Seriously, step one is to get all of the ingredients... every single one of them. **THEN** you can come back home and start preparation

2. **Set a Start Date and, Immediately, Jump into the Modified Diet, Eliminating ALL of The Banned Foods.** I don't want you to just read this book and remain in limbo. Pick the date when you will start the detox program and, without delay, put to practice the cleansing diet that we talked about.

Remember that the body will be undergoing a deep cleansing process and will need as much help as you can give it. Eating light and clean is one of the best ways to attain the very best benefits from your effort. If you keep eating poorly and in excess, then all of the detox in the world will only help marginally. Please... please... please... adjust your diet for at least 10 days before you begin the detox, and maintain it for the 30-day duration.

Believe me, you will lose substantial weight and experience tremendous detoxification. When hunger and/or cravings come around to hassle you, drink two large glasses of water and breathe. Spend time writing about your health-related goals. Fill your mind with the powerful reasons why you want to accomplish this detox cleanse, and in which way will your life be improved with total body detoxification.

The cost of this cleansing process is minimal in comparison to the huge health benefits that you will receive, not to mention added quality years of life!

3. **Dive Into The Detox Program: Make Sure to Follow it as Outlined.** Try not to 'rewrite' my instructions and do them 'your way.' Start with the kidney detox, follow it with the parasite killer remedy and conclude with the liver detox and water enema. Do it in <u>that order</u>. And make sure **NOT** to skip the enema at the end.

Do not exceed the dosages that I have outlined in any of the remedies. Realize that, for the 30 days, your body will be in deep cleansing, healing and repair. Try to get as much rest as you can and do **<u>NOT</u>** force yourself to function at the same levels that you are accustomed. If you get tired easier than usual, that is normal. Give your body a break and be good to yourself.

4. **Stay Close to and Communicate with at least one person that you trust who will support you in this task and not judge.** Any type of detox cleansing is initially going to be challenging, so it helps a lot to have someone standing by to give you a hand and cheer you on. So don't be a Lone Ranger please.

This step is designed to give you ongoing "human" support. Human support will prove invaluable to you during this cleanse.

Go to Fitness Through Fasting's -- <u>Fasting & Detoxification Forum</u> and post messages. Ask for a buddy! Read other people's posts and reach out! You will find many others on the same path. You may even make life-long friends!

5. **Think Hard and Long About What We Talked About Related to Mastering Food, Food Combinations and Getting Active.** As I have said several times, it is absolutely imperative for you to adopt healthy eating habits and a lifestyle that supports your detoxification efforts. It doesn't matter if you have eaten poorly for decades and everyone in your family is overweight. You are a unique and special individual capable of creating your own destiny. Start to make better and healthier decisions for yourself. Get active; find an activity that you enjoy and start doing it at least three times per week for half an hour. I realize that it is tough to change eating and lifestyle habits.

But, in truth, it is tougher to **NOT** change them and have to face adverse health consequences later, don't you think? When tempted to stray, always remember: Nothing Tastes as Good as Thin Feels!

God bless,

ROBERT DAVE JOHNSTON

Volume 3: Lose 30 Pounds in 30 Days (Or More) With Intermittent Fasting & At-Home Coffee Enemas

"From personal experience as well as that of others, you can expect to lose anywhere from 7-10 pounds weekly from intermittent fasting."

Chapter 1:
Rapid Weight Loss &
Detoxification

Without a doubt, the number one, most-asked question I receive about fasting is this
– >

What is the Fastest Way to Lose Weight & Detoxify?

* If I had to narrow it down to two steps, these would be:

1) **Intermittent Fasting**

2) **Home "Coffee" Enemas**

I am assuming that you want to transform your life and health, not just put a little patch on the situation, right? • You want to: Lose weight & cleanse your body of harmful toxins that threaten your health and wellbeing. • Gain knowledge that can **CONTINUALLY** help you maintain optimum weight and health. In think we can agree on those, right? So, let's talk about how to make it happen! :-)

Intermittent Fasting

Intermittent fasting is practiced by many religions around the world. If you are a catholic, for example, you may be familiar with the way "lent" fasting is observed. To be sure, there are many different ways one can practice intermittent fasting.

But I don't want to bombard you with too much information. I want to draw a straight line from where you are now, to where you want to get. To simplify matters, we are going to refer to intermittent fasting as the practice of not eating from 10pm to 6pm each day, for 30 days.

20 Hours of Fasting Daily

This means that you will be fasting 20 hours daily, but will get to have dinner and a snack every night. You can do this for whatever period of time you wish.

However, for our purposes, we are sticking with the 30-day format for **maximum weight loss and detoxification.**

Water Fasting

During the day you will be water fasting. When I say water fasting, I mean that you will be drinking water only. For 20 hours each day during the 30 days, you will eat no solid food, limiting yourself only to water. Very simple, right?

Well, there is much wisdom and power to this practice. While with intermittent fasting the digestive system does not go into total hibernation as it happens during an extended water fast (not eating for more than 72 hours), the body still receives much-needed time to rest from the endless process of digestion. This 'time off' gives the digestive system the opportunity to focus on other important tasks such as detoxification, healing, tissue repair and, of course, rapid weight loss."

Monster Weight Loss

From personal experience as well as that of others, you can expect to lose anywhere from 7-10 pounds weekly from this type of intermittent fasting. I know of some people who have done this fast/detox program and lost in excess of 40, even 50 pounds. I can't guarantee that you will lose that much weight. However, if you follow my instructions in detail, you will lose **A LOT** of weight for sure. :-)

Alright – Let's Go!

Chapter 2:
Cut Out the Junk

If you have been eating poorly and/or excessively, then I strongly advise you to go through a preparation phase of 7-10 days <u>prior to starting</u>. What do I mean by preparation?

Simply this: removing from your diet any and all junk, greasy and sugary foods that you are accustomed to eating. The removal of these toxic foods will send your body into ultimate detoxification and fat-burning mode, so you will lose weight before you even begin fasting.

Furthermore, a lot of the tougher toxins will be processed during those initial preparation days, meaning that the fasting detoxification symptoms will usually be less than if you didn't prepare at all. To keep matters simple, here is a list of the foods that you should avoid for 7-10 days before you start this program.

Banned Foods

*Salt - The foods we eat all have sodium. A healthy adult really has no need for 'salt' except to make the food taste better. When I stopped using salt, I immediately dropped 15 pounds. It was mostly water weight, but it showed me that I was retaining a **LOT** of liquids, and that was greatly due to my abuse of salt and seasonings. Instead of salt, I have become accustomed to seasoning my food with garlic powder (not garlic salt), onion powder (*not onion salt*) and a few of the Ms. Dash no-salt seasonings. I don't even miss salt anymore. I can eat and enjoy food that, in the past, would have been totally bland. My taste buds have readjusted and I feel much better.

* Sugar - absolute trash, toxic to the body... good for nothing - stay away! I could write pages and pages about sugar. I am sure that you yourself can admit that this is one of our greatest (if not our greatest) enemy. I mean it. Enemy. Any prolonged return to sugar will, sooner or later, result in full-blown intoxication of the bloodstream and digestive system. I don't kid myself by thinking that "I'm cured."

I still am susceptible to sugar and to binging. What keeps me free and clean is **NOT** to put sugar into my body... period. I can't draw the same conclusion for you, but I am certain that you probably have your own stories to tell about sugar and how it has affected your weight, life and health.

* **Fried Foods** - Absolute filthy grease fest that leads to obesity and other diseases.

* **Cheese** - Cheese is delicious but is packed with fat. For the time being, steer clear. Later on, once you finish the fast and detox, you can decide what you wish to do.

Don't let the mind start telling you that your 'life is over' because you can't eat this or that. Just **tell the mind to shut up and keep moving forward**. Works like a charm for me.

* **Dairy Products** - dairy has a lot of fat, is high in sugar content and has been known to cause digestive system inflammation. But I'm not totally heartless. Stick to non-fat milk, how's that? Anything above non-fat is banned.

* **Red Meat** - I personally don't have anything against red meat. In fact, I have been known to eat a piece of meat on rare occasion. Right now, we are banning it because it has a lot of fat, and because I want your digestive system to be given easy food to digest. Later on you can have a piece of meat here and there if you want. Right now... it's banned.

* **Alcohol** - Alcohol is packed with empty calories. Calories with **ZERO** nutritional value. And booze turns to sugar. Bad all over. If you drink frequently, cut it down to a minimum. You're doing this for your health and to reach a goal that is important to **YOU**. If you have to go a few days without drinking, your arm is not going to fall off. You'll live. A cup of wine with dinner is fine, but nothing more than that at this juncture.

* **Butter or Margarine** - As they say in New York, "Forget about it!!!" Butter and margarine are pure fat and we don't want it.

* **Fruit Juices** - If you read the label of most orange juice brands, you will see that the sugar content is through the roof.

Yes, it is natural sugar, but sugar nonetheless. You can have one glass of juice in the morning, but you need to water it down 50/50. Drinking straight juice at this phase is basically like injecting blubber directly into your belly. Stay away. Drink veggie juice instead...but make sure that it is the low sodium veggie juice.

*White Enriched Bread - That stuff is like dropping a ball of cement into the stomach. White flour, doughy garbage really is terrible for human health. I was going to ban all breads, but I remembered that the Ezekiel brand (green bag) is actually very good. You can eat one slice here and there as partial replacement to your carbohydrate servings. We'll get into all of that in just a minute.

*Junk Food of ANY Kind - I think that it definitely goes without saying that junk food is out. And not just out for a little while. Hopefully, it is out of your life for good. That crap is like wearing a ball and chain. It enslaves us to cravings that are never satisfied and only get stronger and more violent.

Foods to Limit List:

*Fruits
(Stick To Strawberries or Cantaloupe)
* Tomatoes
* Peas or Corn
* Olive Oil

Starting immediately, eliminate **ALL** of these foods and beverages from your diet... period. This is the beginning of the process. For now, continue to eat whatever else you have been eating **EXCEPT** for the foods that are listed above. I want you to take a full step forward and discontinue eating any and all junk. That's the whole point of our work together, right? To help you achieve measurable improvements in your health. So cut it all out.

Do not eat <u>even a little</u> of them anymore. I mean <u>Nothing</u>, <u>No More</u>, <u>Finito</u>, <u>Nada</u>! You are taking the <u>monumental</u> step of removing **ALL** toxic foods from your diet. I use the word '*monumental*' because, in truth, you are now in the minority. The majority of people live their whole lives and **NEVER** confront their eating behaviors as you are now doing. And since (*hopefully*) you won't be dumping more crap into your belly, the intermittent fasting and coffee enema cleanse will be able to go deep and discharge any hardened debris that hasn't come out via regular vowel movements.

You man now wonder: Ok, so what **CAN** I eat? To answer your question, let me show you my usual menu, which you can use as is, or arrange in similar fashion. The most important part of this preparation phase is that you steer clear of the 'banned foods' listed above. Do that and you will be on your way to amazing results with the actual fast and detox program. Fail to do it, and you will bring upon yourself greater discomfort than you should, and – worse yet – the results will not be optimal. So, please: Follow my instructions as closely as you possibly can. Trust me, I have gone through this countless times and can tell you with certainty that preparation prior to fasting is absolutely indispensable.

Chapter 3:
Sample Pre-Fasting Menu

As I said, you can use this menu exactly as written, or you can match it as close as possible. What matters most, once more, is that you observe the banned foods listed above. Follow this clean diet for at least 7 days before starting with intermittent fasting and coffee enemas. This is the path that will help you yield the best and most measurable results. The good news, however, is that the pre-fasting meal structure still allows you to eat generously; although – of course – there will be restrictions.

Sample Menu:

Breakfast 8:00 AM

1 Cup of Oatmeal with 1 Cup Skim Milk, a Handful of Raisins or Plums
Three Egg Whites mixed with, 3 OZ Ground Turkey
1 Cup of Green Tea with Stevia.

Mid-Morning Snack 10AM

1 Apple or Pear Mixed With One Cup of Nonfat Yogurt (Plain)
OR, ONE Apple, Pear, Banana or Other Fruit

Lunch - Noon

Big salad with lettuce, tomato and other veggies you may like. For dressing, use olive oil (no more than 1 teaspoon) and balsamic vinegar.1 Envelope of Low-Sodium Tuna
1 4OZ Baked Potato or Sweet Potato

Mid-Afternoon Snack 3PM

Same as before - I usually have a piece of fruit mixed with yogurt. At this time in the afternoon, I also drink another cup of green tea.

Green tea has energy-boosting and body-heating properties. It will help to give you a pep as well as calm hunger pangs. In addition to green tea, seltzer water *(sparkling water/club soda)* is great to navigate hunger.

Dinner - 6PM

Six-to-eight ounces of chicken, fish or ground turkey (I like to make turkey patties)
Large salad as the one eaten for lunch. Steamed Broccoli, Cauliflower and Carrots (most supermarkets have prepackaged vegetable combinations that are ready to steam and eat).
4OZ Baked Potato or Sweet Potato **OR** 4OZ of Whole Wheat or Whole Grain Pasta **OR** 4 OZ of Brown Rice.

Evening Snack - 8PM

Big salad with 3OZ Chicken, Fish or Ground Turkey - **No carbohydrates**. A piece of fruit with Non-fat Yogurt. Cup of Chamomile Tea - Chamomile tea is great to drink at night because it will help soothe hunger as well as calm you and get you ready for bed.

Note: You should not eat anything at least two hours prior to turning in, so time the final snack with your bedtime so that there the two-hour window is observed. I usually eat my last snack at around 10pm.

Sometimes I also take one 500 mg tablet of <u>Tryptophan</u> at night to help me sleep. Tryptophan is an awesome amino acid that helps to stabilize mood. At this point I'm done eating for the day and drink only water until 6PM the following evening.

Again ->

NEVER EAT FOR THE LAST TWO HOURS BEFORE YOU GO TO BED.

When the body is at rest, all of the metabolic processes slow down. You won't burn as many calories as you do during the day while you're moving around. When you eat large portions of food shortly before going to bed, many of those calories are directly stored as fat. In addition, rather than healing and restoring, the body spends the night digesting.

The end result, at least for me, is waking up feeling like a truck ran over me. Just slept eight hours, yet I feel tired, lethargic and irritable. **Bottom line**: Eating less than two hours before going to bed is a bad Idea. Tape your mouth shut if you have to. But eat no more!

Chapter 4:
Getting Started

Once you have completed the 7-10 days of preparation, you are ready to jump into the main part of this program. **<u>Do this</u>**:

• Pick the Day that you are going to start. Have your last regular meal the previous evening no later than 9 PM. Do not overeat thinking you are "*stuffing*" for the fast. That will only worsen the hunger pains and detox symptoms. In fact, that is precisely the reason why I asked you to do 7-10 days of preparation, so that your stomach will begin to shrink and start to require less foods to be satisfied.

• Start a **fasting journal** several days before you start. Include detailed writing on how much weight you want to lose and what your general goals are in this process. Write about your ideal body weight and the things you will do once you achieve it. A lot of people balk when I talk to them about starting a journal of any kind. I don't understand why. **Keeping a journal of your goals, progress and challenges is**

one of the most powerful ways to ensure that you'll go the distance and achieve all of your objectives. There is nothing more powerful than reading your own reasons when you feel tired and wish to give up. So, please – do it! :-)

• Start your fast in the **AM** of the chosen day. Drink only water when the hunger pains hit you. Write on your journal if you start to feel angry, irritable or sad. These symptoms are normal and will pass as the days go by.

• If the hunger pains get really bad, try some seltzer/sparkling water with a small twist of lime. If this does not work, then drink more water and your stomach will be satisfied. Write on the fasting journal some more. Remind yourself why you are doing this and stick to your guns. And remind yourself that you will actually get to eat at the end of each day!

• Tell your belly to shut up. You are the boss of your body, not the other way around. Get angry with your stomach and *"literally"* tell it to be quiet and do as it is told. This sounds very silly but it has worked wonders for me. It has taught me that, in the end, I am the one who decides when and what to eat.

• At night, between 6 pm and 8 pm, eat a light meal made up mostly of poultry, fish, vegetables, brown rice and salad. Sugar and fried food of any type are strongly discouraged. Here's the meal that I usually have when I do this type of intermittent fast. It's the same one listed on the sample menu above. Make it as simple as possible so that, when nighttime comes, you don't find yourself wondering what you are going to eat. Plan ahead and make sure that you have everything that you will need to prepare the meals.

Dinner - 6PM

Six ounces of chicken, fish or ground turkey (I like to make turkey patties) Large salad and Steamed Broccoli, Cauliflower and Carrots (*most supermarkets have prepackaged vegetable combinations that are ready to steam and eat*). 4OZ Baked Potato or Sweet Potato OR 4OZ of Whole Wheat or Whole Grain Pasta OR 4 OZ of Brown Rice. For salad dressing, use a small dab of Olive

Oil and a splash of Balsamic Vinegar.

Evening Snack - 8PM

Big salad with 3OZ Chicken, Fish or Ground Turkey - No carbohydrates. A piece of fruit with Non-fat Yogurt. Cup of Chamomile Tea.

As we discussed earlier, please do **NOT** eat anything else after your last snack. The body needs those 12 hours of nightly fasting to process and expel all of the toxins that fasting and coffee enemas will bring to the surface.

• Keep a gallon of water next to your bed. If you wake up hungry in the middle of the night, take a large swig and go back to bed. If your bathroom happens to be next to the kitchen and you have to go, then go with blinders on - DO **NOT** by any means enter the kitchen for any reason whatsoever!

In The Morning

• Upon rising, have a large glass of water to stimulate the bowels. Record on your journal how you are feeling physically and emotionally. If you have any vivid or strange dreams, write about them.

The release of large amounts of toxins into the bloodstream, as it occurs when fasting, can sometimes cause strange dreams. It is normal and will pass.

Fast the entire day following the steps described above.

• Carry out the coffee enema (*outlined below*) three times per week for the first two weeks, twice for the third week and once during the final week of the fast.

Monday, Wednesdays and Fridays are my personal choices.

• It is best to do the enema in the morning or, second best, at night **BEFORE** you break the fast with the evening meal.

• Make sure to read the instructions below several times so that you can learn to listen to your body and follow the protocol in a way that is best for your particular makeup and condition.

• On the last day of the fast, break it in the evening as usual. Incorporate coffee enemas and 24-hour water fasting into your lifestyle at least <u>once per month</u>.

• Most of all, do not return to consumption of damaging foods. There's nothing worse than going through all of this work and sacrifice and then throwing a wrench in it by resuming a poor diet. It is my hope that, after this process, you will want to make permanent eating habit and lifestyle changes so that you can keep the benefits long term!

All told, you can lose from 30 to 50 pounds with this system, not to mention that you'll be ridding your body of disease-causing toxins & parasites.

Let's take a look at some of the detox symptoms that you may experience while fasting and cleansing.

Chapter 5:
Detox Symptoms

Headaches – This one is especially marked for coffee drinkers, but is also the case for persons who consume large amounts of sugar and alcohol. This symptom can really take a person out of commission. A lot of my colleagues call me a heretic for saying this, but if you need to take a couple of ibuprofen tablets to ease the pain, then so be it. Usually two tablets will do the trick. But don't take more than four daily. You may need to go through a little pain and discomfort. The good news is that headaches rarely last more than 72 hours, if that.

Dizziness – The body is not used to being deprived of eating whatever it wants and will go through dizzy spells, particularly during the first 11 days. The best solution for dizziness is to move slowly and get as much rest as your daily schedule allows.

Difficulty Performing Basic Tasks – Since you aren't consuming solid food, it will take some time for the body to adjust. You will more than likely feel very weak and may have trouble getting around - particularly during the first 10-14 days. If you slow down and work on focusing on the individual tasks you are performing, this symptom can be overcome. It is important for you to realize that your body is going through a transition. You must move slowly and not try to push yourself too hard. You may not be able to function at the same capacity as you are accustomed. Fine. Slow down and give the body time to work on your behalf.

Weakness means that you need to be extra careful when walking around, and especially when getting up from a sitting position. Avoid harsh and/or abrupt movements. Move slowly, watch your step closely and always have something that you can hang on to if you suddenly feel like you are fainting. This is good advice.

One time I totally hit the deck because I got up to quickly from a chair. I missed the corner of the wall by centimeters, but still hit myself quite hard on the floor. This is about improving our health, not about getting hurt. Please be careful. I mean it. Be careful.

Pulsating Hunger Pains that disappear and then re-emerge throughout the day. For some persons, hunger is monstrous in the morning. But for the vast majority, the hunger troll shows up mostly at night. In short, hunger will always be a part of our lives, and it is our task to master it rather than allow it to enslave us as it **CAN AND WILL** if we let it.

In my case, hunger was very strong in the first week to 10 days of intermittent fasting, and then I found myself getting used to always being 'a little' hungry. After a while, I loved it because I began to feel more alert, more energetic, optimistic... I slept better. I actually **SLEPT THROUGH THE NIGHT** and woke up feeling terrific.

Before the fast, I constantly woke up at night to urinate, or like a raving lunatic wanting to raid the fridge. After a while, I would go to sleep at 11PM, close my eyes and, when I opened them, it was 6AM! For me, this was nothing less than a total miracle. And I felt great... refreshed and ready to go! All of that just from getting used to eating less and being a little hungry.

Much better than getting stuffed like a boar as I used to.

Bad Breath, Metallic Taste in Mouth, White Sticky Film on Tongue – These are all good indications that your body is eliminating toxicity.

Most of these symptoms pass after 14 days (on average). Bad Breath, I suggest that you get sugarless mints and keep them handy until the process ends.

Metallic Taste In the Mouth usually means that there are excessive (and toxic) heavy metals accumulated in your system.

I recall having this constant sulfur and 'steel' taste in my mouth for about a week.

White Sticky Film on the Tongue can be disgusting, but it's a sign that the body is cleansing. For these symptoms, the best thing you can do is to keep drinking a lot of water. Make sure to brush your teeth regularly. Keep a travel toothbrush with you if you spend a lot of time out. Mouthwash is also helpful.

Diarrhea or Constipation – All of the fecal matter adhered to your colon will either start gushing out in diarrhea or incite short-term constipation. I know that this is disgusting, but it happens. If you have eaten poorly for a long time, or have simply abused sugar or fat, your body may respond to the water fast by starting to expel all of the toxic filth in this fashion.

If **Diarrhea** Strikes, simply continue to follow the fast as outlined. Should it become severe, see your pharmacist and ask him or her for an over-the-counter recommendation.

Continue with the intermittent fast. Fasting is a shock to the body, but it will finally get the message and react favorably to what you are doing. If you have diarrhea, make sure to keep yourself hydrated.

Make it a point to drink at least one gallon of water daily. Stay close to a bathroom at all times. If you go out, make sure that you are always aware where the nearest restroom is. Seriously, you want to get to the toilet promptly anytime you need to.

If **Constipation** is The Case, visit your local pharmacy and ask your pharmacist about a stool softener. I personally use a herbal laxative called Herbs & Prunes. It works like a charm every time and is not harsh on my stomach. Take one tablet to start. Do not exceed four tablets in one day. But do this only if you fail to eliminate anything for at least three days. Give your body enough time to do it on its own.

Irritability / Mood Swings – If you have ever seen The Flintstones, you may remember Fred walking around growling on the episode where he is placed on a diet. Sooooo, be prepared to be a little *"short-fused"* during this time fasting and cleansing. Be aware that you will not be as patient as you normally would. Tell your loved ones not to take it personally if - initially - you are less social that what they are accustomed. This is normal and will pass.

Facial Puffiness & Feeling Bloated – This symptom is much more marked for persons who consume large amounts of salt and/or sugar. I personally was bloated to the max like the Stay Puft Marshmallow man.

So being puffy was nothing new. I looked like somebody had stuck huge balloons on my cheeks. It was hideous. Fasting took care of that and my face today is that of a normal human being rather than a cartoon character.

That is a lot of symptoms, but rarely does **ONE** person experience them all. And remember, they will subside and mostly pass after approximately 14 days. Continue to surrender to the process and stay put. Let the body do what it does best. Your body knows how to take care of you. Your body and digestive system thank you for this break. Your body is loyal and noble ... it is unleashing amazing weight loss and healing power even as we speak. All you have to do is hang on and let the process run its course.

Chapter 6:
Coffee Enemas

Yes, you heard right – I said Coffee enemas. This, without a doubt, is one of the most powerful detoxification tools I have discovered in my years as a fasting coach and practitioner. Caffeine incites stimulation of the digestive system which in turn induces what can often be dramatic elimination of toxic, hardened feces & parasites adhered to the walls of the colon.

If you look at the picture above, you can see the different conditions that can emerge when the colon is overloaded with toxins. And, trust me, you will be eliminating a lot of gunk. Even if you have eaten a clean diet, it is possible that you may still have substantial waste accumulated. One man that I know eliminated pounds and pounds of undigested meat that was rotting in his colon!

Typically I am asked: *"Well, what is the difference between drinking coffee and a coffee enema?"*

Answer: "Drinking coffee often induces a bowel movement. This, effect, however is much deeper and thorough **when the coffee is injected directly into the colon rather than just as a beverage**. It is a very powerful colon detoxification technique."

Gross!

Now, when I start to talk about feces, parasites and enemas, many persons rapidly balk and become *"grossed out,"* indicating that they are not interested in anything that has to do with "rectal insertion." They are, in essence, horrified by the prospect. You would think one is asking them to sever a limb or something.

My response is always the same: "Well, would you rather be a little grossed out and rid your body of these derelict parasites and toxins **NOW**, or would you prefer to deal with them **LATER** in a hospital bed or – god forbid – with a life-threatening illness?"

If you are one of these persons, I hope this response helps to put things in perspective. Believe me, whatever feeling of *"grossness"* you feel is small in comparison to the huge health benefits this practice can offer. Ok, so how is this done?

Do this: Go to your local pharmacy and/or health store and purchase a One Gallon Enema Kit at the very minimum. The link above takes you to Amazon.com so you can see what I am talking about.

In addition, purchase a bag of surgical gloves, as well as some Vaseline or other lubricant **AND** rubbing alcohol. One you have the enema kit, gloves, alcohol and lubricant on hand, it's time to prepare the coffee solution and get started.

Preparing the Coffee Solution

In terms of which type of coffee to use, the truth is that it doesn't really matter so long as it is caffeinated, of course. I use either Maxwell House or Café Bustelo. They both do the job quite well. But you can safely use whatever coffee you are used to drinking. What we're after is the caffeine in the liquid. I have not found any particular brand to work better than another.

Follow this step-by-step-approach:

• The night before, brew at least 2 full pots of coffee – equivalent to 12 cups in most coffee makers. Use 10 table spoons of coffee for each brewing.

• Place each yield of coffee in a large soup pan for cooling. If you don't have a large pan, you may need to use several smaller ones. The point is that you pour the coffee into a separate recipient for cooling.

• Take at least 3 empty water gallons and fill each *"halfway"* with filtered or purified water. I strongly discourage the use of tap water.

Fill the rest of the gallon with the cooled coffee. Continue this process until you have filled at least <u>three</u> gallons of the coffee/water mixture. This should last you one week.

Getting It Done

• When you are ready, go to your bathroom and place various towels on the floor next to the door, as well as two pillows. I also bring in a <u>portable radio and put on soothing music for relaxat</u>ion.

• Assemble the enema bag with the enclosed hook for the top, the hose and "*inserter*" at the bottom. Make sure the enema "lock" is closed. Pour some water on the enema bag and make sure that it is not leaking and that the lock is properly in place.

• Many enema hoses have various "lock" positions that go from zero, to small, to large releases of liquid. Get acquainted with the one you have and learn how to go from little to more water with each different lock position. Learn exactly where the "total lock" position is.

• Play with the hose for a few minutes until you feel comfortable with it and understand how to regulate the levels of liquid that it releases. If the one you have only goes from lock to release, observe the amount of liquid that comes out when it is open.

The point is, see what you are working with **NOW**. Once you are on the floor and using it, you do not want any surprises.

• When all looks good, dump the "test" water and fill the enema bag with the coffee/water mixture. Carry the enema bag to the bathroom through the plastic hook at the top (*enclosed with the enema*).

• Hang the enema bag in the bathroom door knob. I use the door knob because it grants enough slack between the hose and body.

Experiment in your bathroom and find the most comfortable location for the bag. Make sure the enema bag is steady and that it will not fall wherever you decide to place it.

• Next, wash your hands thoroughly with hot water. Use <u>germ-killing bar or liquid soap</u>. Scrub all the way up your forearms like a surgeon before surgery.

• Turn <u>off</u> all telephones and, if you live with others, make sure that you inform them not to disturb you.

• Next, put on the sterilized plastic gloves. Get the Vaseline and lubricate the "inserter" tip of the enema.

• Lay down sideways on the floor, your head on one of the pillows and your back facing the enema bag. Depending on which side you lay, grab the inserter with your free hand. It is now time to do the deed.

• Slowly spread some lubricant around your rectum. Little by little, insert the tip of the enema inside of you. Take your time. Do not force it in. If it feels dry and painful, take it out and put more lubricant. Repeat this process until you are able to insert it without undue pain.

• Once in, reach to the enema bag lock. Take a deep breath and release the lock so that it starts to let out the smallest amount of the coffee/water mixture. You will feel the cool liquid start to enter your belly.

• Let the liquid continue to enter your colon for at least ten seconds. Lock the hose and make sure the surge of liquid has stopped.

• Begin to massage your stomach from different angles. At this point you may or may not get the urge to eliminate. If you do, try to hold it - if you can. If not, then go ahead and eliminate.

• If you **CAN** hold it, then "open" the lock again for another ten seconds, this time so that it releases a larger amount of the coffee/water mixture.

• Once you feel your colon is pretty full of the mixture, remove the inserter from your rectum, wrap it in toilet paper and set it aside.

•Lay face up with one pillow under your head and another one under your lower back.

Massaging the Belly

It is now that the real work begins. Spend as much time as possible massaging your stomach with both hands –> covering the left, right, bottom and upper parts of your abdomen. Pay close attention to your liver. Let the music sink in and visualize toxins, parasites and hardened feces being expelled from your body. Take as much time as needed in this process. Really, really work it!

For some persons with large levels of toxicity, the evacuation process can be dramatic and almost immediate. If that is the case for you, go ahead and eliminate. You may feel cramps in your stomach and some abdomen pain. This is fairly normal for most people. Make sure to look at the discharge once you are done. What color is it? Is it really dark or even black? If so, then it is likely that you are making good progress.

If at any time you see blood in the stool, stop the enema immediately and go see your doctor at once! Repeat this method until the mixture in the enema bag is consumed. If the evacuation does not instantly come, persist with the massage. If there is still no discharge, go ahead and eliminate and repeat the process. You may have very hardened or stubborn buildup in your bowels.

Chapter 7:
Take Your Time

For me, the process was very slow. I actually would fill my colon with the mixture, get up and go about other business around the house, keeping the liquid inside of me for several hours at a time.

It may take time for the dregs of fecal matter to soften and be expelled. Don't give up! So, if you are the type who is slow to discharge, get up and do something else. But please, stay close to a bathroom at all times! Let's avoid embarrassing accidents!

Adjusting the Coffee Mix

Use up the entire contents of the enema bag during the day. I recommend you do the whole bag in one session. But, if you are pressed for time, **it is okay to do part in the morning and the rest at night – so long as you do not use the same mixture**! Dump any unused mixture at once; do not store it for later use, please. If you find that the current mixture is not working, prepare another one with more coffee. Go from, say, 10 tablespoons of coffee per pot to 15.

Keep trying until you find your magic number. For some people who are obese and highly toxic, as many as 20 tablespoons of coffee per pot (or more) may be required. Take it slow and continue the process until you find the right formula for you. But do not overdo it with the coffee! It is best to start low and go up gradually. If you add too much coffee, you may get very painful and uncomfortable cramps. Don't make it any harder than it has to be, please!

When you are done, make sure to wash the inserter with hot water and soap, **AND** dip it into a small cup filled with rubbing alcohol. Do this with the gloves still on. Wash the enema bag in warm water with the hose "open" so that it cleanses the inside of it as well. Hang it to dry. I hang mine in the shower curtain bar.

Be very thorough with the inserter and make sure it is painstakingly clean and sterilized. Once done, wrap it again in toilet paper and put it away with the enema bag as described below. Make sure you store the enema kit where others will **NOT** have access to it.

NEVER share the inserter with anybody else no matter how clean it is. In fact, don't share the enema bag at all.

Let each family member interested in fasting and cleansing purchase one of their own. Pick up the towels from the floor and put them in the washer, along with the pillow cases from the pillows you used during the process.

Once the enema bag is dry, I recommend you store it in a "zip-lock" bag along with the inserter. That way your kit will not be exposed to dust, germs or any type of dirt. If you need to mop the bathroom because some liquid spilled, do so **BUT** keep the gloves on.

Bleach the bathroom floor as well as the toilet. When you are done, THEN remove the gloves and throw them out. Go through the initial hand-washing process again and finalize by sprinkling them with rubbing alcohol. Allow hands to air dry. If you have children, **DO NOT** dispose of the gloves by simply throwing them on top of the garbage pail. One of the little-ones may reach in and retrieve them! On the next session, wash each part of the kit thoroughly and again sterilize the inserter with rubbing alcohol.

The bottom line is this: with intermittent fasting combined with coffee enemas, you will experience very rapid weight loss as well as the deep cleansing of your bowels.

This regimen is extremely powerful. If you take the time to really get good at it, you will truly revolutionize your health. It may take some time to see the huge results that you seek, but if you are persistent, I can assure you that they will come.

Be patient and kind to your body, and it will pay you back in spades – guaranteed. In addition to discharging a lot of toxic muck from your bowels, you will start to feel lighter, more energetic, with greater mental energy and clarity.

I know of people who found relief from chronic depression and other mental illnesses via coffee enemas and intermittent fasting. If you stick to the plan for the 30 days, tremendous things will come to pass in your life and health. To finalize, here's a motivational message that I want you to keep in mind as you move forward.

Chapter 8:
The Challenge of Detoxification

If you stumbled and were not able to complete the entire fast/cleansing, please don't worry. Yes, I know – it is a tough call. But it is not impossible. If you carried out the diet menu as outlined (I strongly encourage you to do so), then you now have a very good idea of the symptoms to expect when you try again.

So... just because you fell short of the goal and were unable to complete the fast/cleanse in one or multiple attempts, that does not mean that you failed. Such distinction is crucial because it is at this point that many give up.

They feel that going the distance is too hard and not feasible. Nothing is further from the truth. It may take a few attempts, but if you continue and not give up, you will make amazing progress.

I was a complete disaster; obese, a food

addict, depressed and suicidal... yet after some tries I **DID** complete the 30-day fast/cleanse. I would dare to say that I owe my life to it. So there is no way that you can fail.

You are continuing to learn and position yourself for breakthrough. This process is challenging but highly rewarding. So do not be discouraged. Progress, not perfection – is the key!

Keep the Journal Alive

Write, write and write as much as you can! Keep putting your thoughts and feelings on paper. Read this book several times until you feel that you have fully internalized the material.

If you truly are committed to change and find yourself struggling, then **it is fine to move at your own pace**. Stick to the program and keep working.

Try, try again. Take notes and learn from your mistakes. Your desire / willingness to change **WILL** help you to produce the breakthrough you want **IF** you stick to it.

You can do it!
When tempted to stray, always remember:
Nothing Tastes as Good as Thin Feels!

God bless and Godspeed,

ROBERT DAVE JOHNSTON

Grab The Entire Collection:

Volume 1: The 'Permanent Weight Loss' Diet

Volume 2: The Intermittent Fasting Weight Loss Formula

Volume 3: How to Lose 30 Pounds (Or More) In 30 Days with Juice Fasting

Volume 4: Lose The Belly Fat Fast, And For Good!

Volume 5: Lose the Emotional Baggage: Transform Your Mind & Spirit with Fasting

Volume 6: How to Break a Fast (or Diet) and Keep the Weight Off

Volume 7: Compilation Volumes 1-6 -> Get All 5 For The Price Of 3!

Also by Robert Dave Johnston:

How to Lose Weight & Keep it Off by Transforming the Mind & Behaviors

Volume 1: How to Build a Rock-Solid Foundation That Supports Long-Term Weight Loss

Volume 2: How to Lose Weight & Keep it Off By Reprogramming The Subconscious Mind

Volume 3: How to Beat Diet Hunger and Junk Food Cravings

Volume 4: How to Escape the Diet "Time Trap" and Succeed in Weight Loss

Volume 5: How to Cheat on Your Diet (And Get Away With It)

Volume 6, Compilation: All 5 for the Price Of 3

Also By Robert Dave Johnston:

Detoxify Your Body, Lose Weight, Get Healthy & Transform Your Life

Volume 1- The 10-Day 'At Home' Colon Cleansing Formula

Volume 2- The 30-Day Kidney, Parasite & Liver Detox Weight Loss Method

Volume 3- Lose Weight Fast & Detoxify With Intermittent Fasting & At-Home Coffee Enemas

Volume 4 - Compilation: Get All 3 For The Price Of 2! Detoxify Your Body, Lose Weight, Get Healthy & Transform Your Life - Volumes 1-3

Don't forget to check the articles and growing health community at: FitnessThroughFasting.com

www.ingramcontent.com/pod-product-compliance
Lightning Source LLC
Chambersburg PA
CBHW030446290526

45786CB00001B/464